Special Tests for
Orthopedic
Examination

SPECIAL TESTS FOR ORTHOPEDIC EXAMINATION

Jeff G. Konin, MEd, ATC, MPT
Delaware Technical & Community College
Georgetown, DE

Denise L. Wiksten, PhD, ATC
The Department of Exercise and Nutritional Sciences
San Diego State University
San Deigo, CA

Jerome A. Isear, Jr., MS, PT, ATC
Carolinas Physical Therapy Associates
Charlotte, NC

SLACK Incorporated, 6900 Grove Road, Thorofare, New Jersey 08086

Publisher: John H. Bond
Editorial Director: Amy E. Drummond
Creative Director: Linda Baker
Copyright © 1997 by SLACK Incorporated

Printed in the United States of America

Konin, Jeff G.
    Special tests for orthopedic examination/Jeff G. Konin, Denise
Wiksten, Jerome A. Isear.
            p. cm.
        ISBN 1-55642-351-9
        1. Physical orthopedic tests.
I. Wiksten, Denise. II. Isear, Jerome A. III. Title.
        [DNLM: 1. Musculoskeletal Diseases--diagnosis--handbooks.
Articular--handbooks. WE 39 K82s 1997]
RD734.5.P58K66 1997
616.7'0754--dc21
DNLM/DLC
for Library of Congress   97-21469

Published by: SLACK Incorporated
                 6900 Grove Road
                 Thorofare, NJ 08086-9447 USA
                 Telephone: 609-848-1000
                 Fax: 609-853-5991
Contact SLACK Incorporated for more information about other books in
this field or about the availability of our books from distributors outside
the United States.

Last digit is print number: 10 9 8 7 6 5 4 3 2 1

Dedication

To Gina, for sharing the ingredients that have made the recipe for life most appetizing.

Jeff G. Konin

To my parents, who have never stopped believing in me. To Dave Perrin and Joe Gieck, for their continued inspiration and direction. To Eric, for his never-ending support and encouragement throughout this project and my career.

Denise L. Wiksten

To my parents, who taught me the true meaning of perseverence. To Dave Perrin, for believing in me and affording me the opportunity to excel.

Jerome A."Jai" Isear, Jr.

Table of Contents

Acknowledgments

The successful completion of this book could not have been accomplished without the hard work and determination of a number of individuals. We would like to express our sincere thanks to Greg Hockman and Holly Priano for graciously posing as subjects for the many photographs. Also to Robin Reed, whose creativity and photography helped us to illustratively explain so many challenging examination techniques. In addition, we appreciate the encouragement that our respected employers, Delaware Technical and Community College, San Diego State University, and Carolinas Physical Therapy Associates, have given us to pursue professional endeavors.

Most importantly, we are indebted to Amy Drummond and SLACK Incorporated, who believed in the three of us and this project. Ideas are like rivers; with momentum, they lead to the oceans of opportunity. The receptiveness, acceptance, cooperation, and nurturing of this book by the professionals of SLACK Incorporated have led to an alternative guide for which members of the health care field can refer to as they seek the necessary tools to improve upon their current level of clinical competency.

Foreword

The physical examination is a critical component of any orthopedic evaluation process. Tests and measurements are used to identify the status of one's range of motion, strength, flexibility, and inert/non-inert structures. As such, a host of special tests must be performed in order to fine-tune the physical examination and ultimately accept or refute a hypothetical diagnosis that may emerge from the subjective and observational portions of the evaluation process. Special tests are essentially designed to isolate specific structures during the evaluation process.

Special Tests for Orthopedic Examination is a unique and valuable reference guide designed for athletic trainers, physical therapists, family physicians, and other health care professionals who provide care for those individuals with orthopedic injuries. Featuring special orthopedic examination techniques, this book is organized in a manner such that the reader can rapidly turn to the description and illustration of a test reflecting a specific location of the body. The summaries of the most commonly performed special tests are clear and concise. The reader is taken through the steps of performing each special test, including subject and examiner positioning, actions, indications, and special considerations. The text is complimented by well over 200 photographs further illustrating the correct technique for each test.

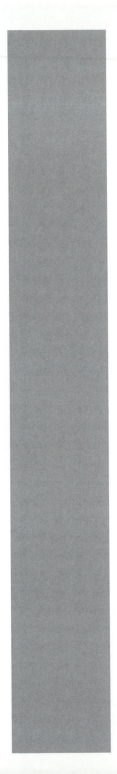

This book will help athletic training, physical therapy, and other allied medical students learn to perform thorough injury evaluations and accurately interpret their findings. It is important to note that special tests are merely one part of an orthopedic examination, and that this book is not intended to replace classroom textbooks that include discussion of injury evaluation. Rather, it is a pocket guide that will help students apply what they have learned in the classroom to clinical and field experiences.

Jeff Konin, Denise Wiksten, and Jai Isear have done a remarkable job of compiling information in one book that will help the student and clinician thoroughly and accurately assess orthopedic injuries, regardless of setting. Wise use of this book will enhance one's clinical examination skills and ultimately improve the quality of care provided to those with orthopedic injuries. Without question, *Special Tests for Orthopedic Examination* is a welcomed addition to the orthopedic-based classrooms, professions, and work-sites.

Craig R. Denegar, PhD, ATC, PT

Preface

An orthopedic physical examination is performed by health care professionals to confirm or reject an injury diagnosis. The injury evaluation process is structured in an orderly and progressive fashion. Following a traumatic injury, the clinician must rule out any instability that may be life threatening or lead to further injury. Once an individual is stabilized, the injury evaluation process follows a survey of questions, observations, and techniques that help to differentiate injured tissue from non-injured tissue. This process includes the performance of special tests. Special tests are designed to stress specific structures and isolate damaged tissue. They are conducted near the end of the examination process and are considered a very specific physical examination technique. Proper execution of special tests will provide valuable information about the specific structure involved and the extent of tissue damage. It is important for clinicians to be proficient and up-to-date in the performance of special tests. Many injury evaluation textbooks include special test performance. However, clinicians have lacked the opportunity to consult a comprehensive, yet simple to understand, quick reference guide that primarily includes orthopedic special test techniques.

Special Tests for Orthopedic Examination is designed as a unique and valuable reference manual for family physicians, athletic trainers, physical therapists, and other health care professionals who provide primary care for sports related and non-athletic orthopedic injuries. The book specifically presents a comprehensive list of special tests used during an orthopedic physical examination. The special tests are organized by regions of the body so the reader can easily reference a particular test. The reader is guided through the mechanics of performing each test followed by the interpretation and significance of a positive test result. The text is clear and concise and is complimented by photographs illustrating the proper subject and clinician positioning. It should be noted that the intent of this book is to assist in the performance of special tests, and not to cover the techniques of performing a complete orthopedic physical examination. The special tests in this book should be used as an adjunct to other orthopedic examination processes and techniques.

This book will also serve as a complimentary text to other textbooks on injury evaluation for students in athletic training, physical therapy, and other allied orthopedic professions. The book will help students learn to perform special tests and accurately interpret their findings. It is a handy pocket guide for students in the classroom and clinical environments.

It is hoped that *Special Tests for Orthopedic Examination* will serve students in orthopedic health professions as well as certified or licensed orthopedic professionals, and will be a valuable resource for the evaluation of orthopedic injuries.

SECTION 1

Head

Cranial Nerve Assessment

TEST POSITIONING:
The positioning of the subject may vary according to the nerve being tested.

ACTION:
The examiner's action will vary according to the cranial nerve being tested.

POSITIVE FINDING:
The absence, delay, or asymmetry of a response indicates possible involvement of the particular nerve that is being individually tested.

SPECIAL CONSIDERATIONS/COMMENTS:
The examiner should assess the individual function of all structures (ie, muscle) to distinguish between neurological and muscular integrity.

CRANIAL NERVE I (OLFACTORY)

Chief Function: Smell.

Test: The examiner places an object that possesses a strong, identifiable odor just under the nasal area of the subject in an attempt to assess the subject's ability to perceive the odor. An ammonia capsule is typically used for this test (Figure 1A).

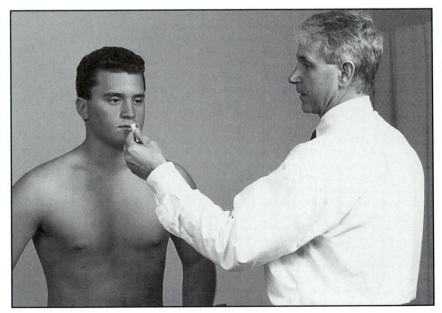

FIGURE 1A

HEAD

CRANIAL NERVE II (OPTIC)

Chief Function: Vision.

Test: The examiner asks the subject to identify objects within view and to clarify what the subject actually sees (Figure 1B).

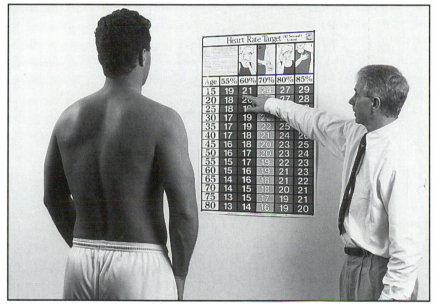

FIGURE 1B

CRANIAL NERVE III (OCULOMOTOR)

Chief Function: Voluntary motor control of levator palpebrae, superior, medial and inferior recti, inferior oblique eye muscles.

Test: The examiner asks the subject to elevate the eyelid and elevate, depress, and adduct the eye (Figure 1C).

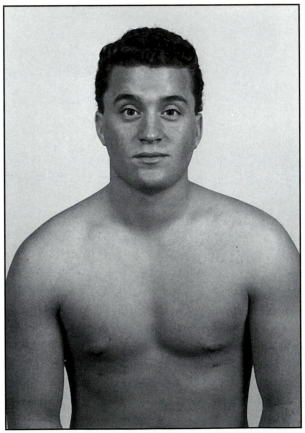

FIGURE 1C

CRANIAL NERVE IV (TROCHLEAR)

Chief Function: Voluntary motor control of superior oblique eye muscle.

Test: The examiner asks the subject to elevate the eye (Figure 1D).

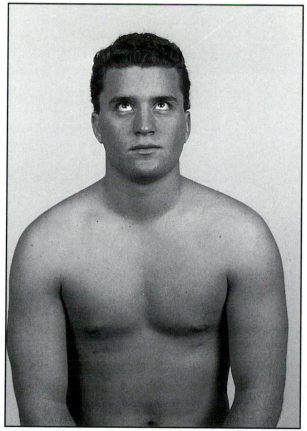

FIGURE 1D

CRANIAL NERVE V (TRIGEMINAL)

Chief Function: Sensation of touch and pain on the skin of the face, mucous membranes of the nose, sinuses, mouth, and anterior tongue. Voluntary motor control of the muscles of mastication.

Test: Sensory: The examiner assesses the subject's ability to perceive touch along the skin of the face (Figure 1E).
Motor: The examiner asks the subject to perform the motions of elevation (Figure 1F), depression (Figure 1G), protrusion, retrusion, and lateral deviation (Figure 1H) of the mandible.

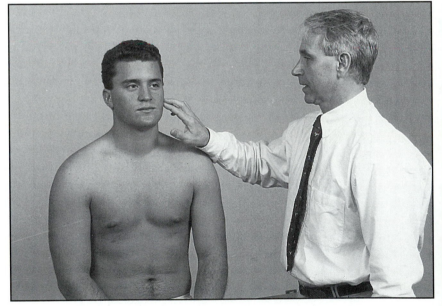

FIGURE 1E

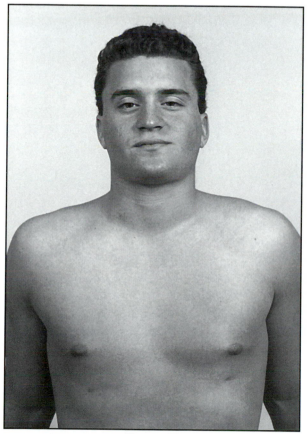

FIGURE 1F

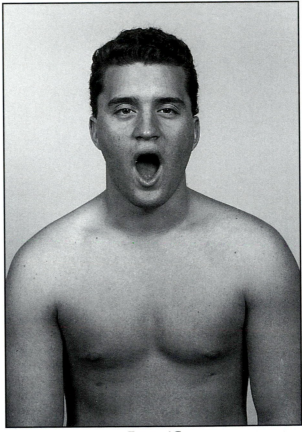

FIGURE 1G

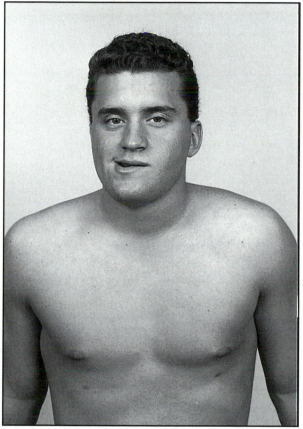

FIGURE 1H

CRANIAL NERVE VI (ABDUCENS)

Chief Function: Voluntary motor control of the lateral rectus muscle of the eye.

Test: The examiner asks the subject to abduct the eye (Figure 1I).

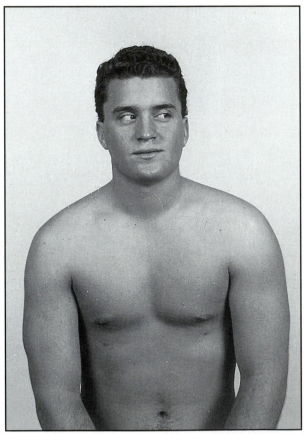

FIGURE 1I

CRANIAL NERVE VII (FACIAL)

Chief Function: Taste along the anterior portion of the tongue. Voluntary motor control of facial muscles.

Test: Sensory: The examiner assesses the subject's ability to distinguish identifiable tasting objects with the anterior portion of the tongue (Figure 1J).

Motor: The examiner can ask the subject to perform any of the following movements:
- elevation, adduction, or depression of the eyebrow
- closure of the eyelid (Figure 1K)
- dilation and constriction of the nasal
- closure of the mouth
- closure and protrusion of the lips (Figure 1L).

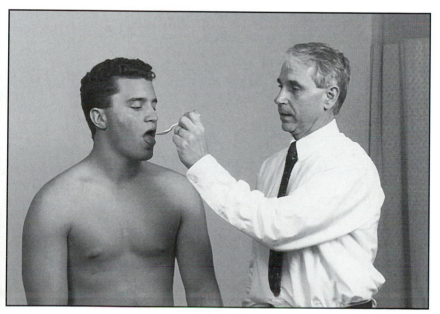

FIGURE 1J

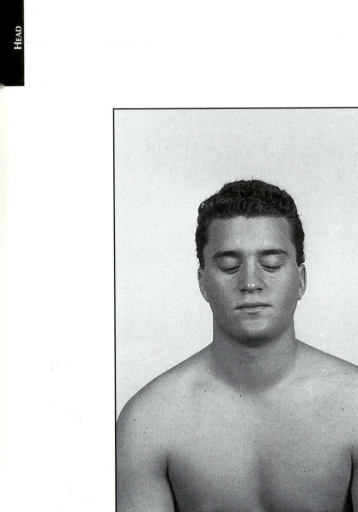

FIGURE 1K

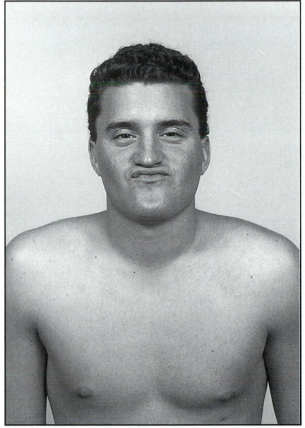

FIGURE 1L

CRANIAL NERVE VIII (VESTIBULOCOCHLEAR)

Chief Function: Hearing and balance via the ear.

Test: The examiner asks the subject to stand with eyes closed and no support in order to assess the subject's balance (Figure 1M).

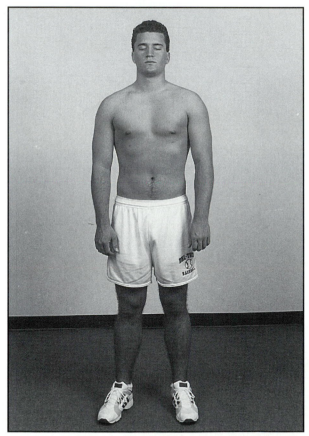

FIGURE 1M

CRANIAL NERVE IX (GLOSSOPHARYNGEAL)

Chief Function: Sensation of touch and pain on the posterior portion of the tongue and pharynx. Taste on the posterior portion of the tongue. Voluntary motor control of some muscles of the pharynx.

Test: Sensory: The examiner assesses the subject's ability to distinguish identifiable tasting objects with the posterior portion of the tongue (Figure 1N).
Motor: The examiner assesses the subject's ability to swallow.

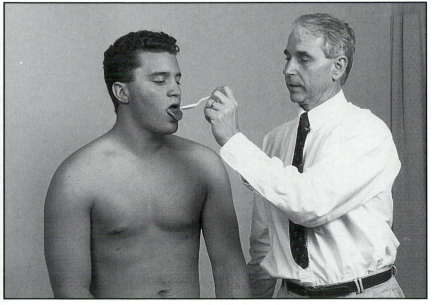

FIGURE 1N

CRANIAL NERVE X (VAGUS)

Chief Function: Sensation of touch and pain of the pharynx, larynx, and bronchi. Autonomic muscle control of the thoracic and abdominal viscera.

Test: The examiner assesses the functioning of the subject's abdominal and thoracic viscera.

CRANIAL NERVE XI (ACCESSORY)

Chief Function: Voluntary motor control of the sternocleidomastoid and trapezius muscles.

Test: The examiner asks the subject to shrug the shoulders (Figure 10).

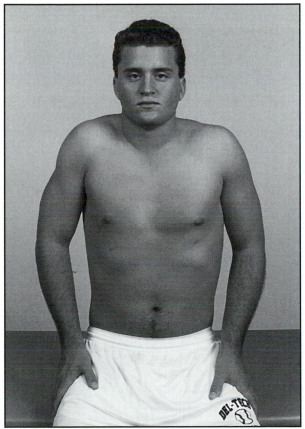

FIGURE 1O

CRANIAL NERVE XII (HYPOGLOSSAL)

Chief Function: Voluntary motor control of the muscles of the tongue.

Test: The examiner asks the subject to protrude the tongue (Figure 1P).

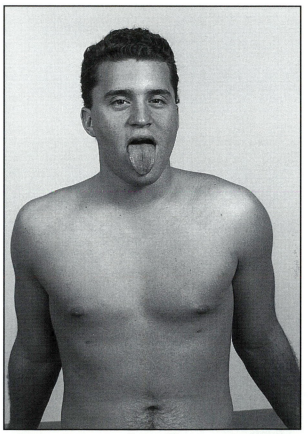

FIGURE 1P

Rhomberg Test

TEST POSITIONING:
The subject stands with eyes closed, feet together, and arms at sides (Figure 2).

ACTION:
Observe the subject's ability to resist postural swaying and/or loss of balance.

POSITIVE FINDING:
Significant postural sway, a loss of balance, or the inability to stand with the eyes closed is indicative of a cerebral injury.

SPECIAL CONSIDERATIONS/COMMENTS:
For highly skilled individuals, this test should be repeated using single leg balance for more of a challenge.

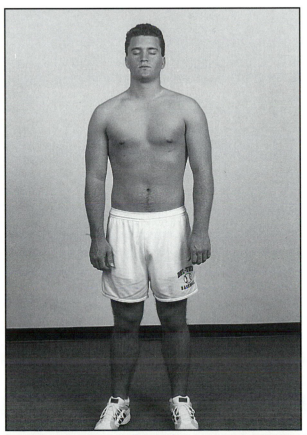

FIGURE 2

Glasgow Coma Scale

TEST POSITIONING:
Subject will most likely be lying on the ground. The examiner must determine the subject's level of consciousness as soon as possible; therefore, the examiner must be quickly position himself next to the subject.

ACTION:
For each of the three following responses, a number is given according to the type of positive response listed below.

1. Determine eye response.
    4   Are the eyes open?
    3   Do the eyes open in response to verbal communication?
    2   Do the eyes open in response to painful stimulation?
    1   Is there no eye response?

2. Determine motor response.
    6   Does the subject obey verbal motor commands (ie, wiggle toes)?
    5   When a painful stimulus is applied, can the subject localize the pain?
    4   When a painful stimulus is applied, does the subject withdraw from the stimulus?
    3   When a painful stimulus is applied, does the subject present decorticate rigidity (ie, upper extremities are extended, internally rotated, and plantar flexed)?
    2   When a painful stimulus is applied, does the subject present decerebrate rigidity (ie, upper extremities are rigidly extended, adducted, and pronated; lower extremities are extended, internally rotated, and plantar flexed)?
    1   Is there no motor response?

3. Determine verbal response.
    5   Is the subject oriented and conversing with examiner?
    4   Is the subject disoriented but still conversing?
    3   Is the subject using inappropriate words?
    2   Is the subject making incomprehensible sounds?
    1   Is there no verbal response?

POSITIVE FINDING:

Any score less than 15 is considered positive. Level of impairment is scaled as follows:

    12 or greater: mild head injury
    9 to 11: moderate head injury
    8 or less: serious head injury.

SPECIAL CONSIDERATIONS/COMMENTS:

1. When assessing motor response, it is important to avoid asking the subject to squeeze something such as your finger or an object. This may produce a reflex grasp and would indicate a false positive response to a verbal motor command.

2. Be certain that "no motor response" is not due to a spinal cord injury; this may produce a false positive.

3. Altered motor response that is unilateral may indicate a specific focal injury.

4. Presence of decorticate rigidity indicates injury above the red nucleus; presence of decerebrate rigidity indicates injury to the brain stem.

5. Head injuries can be considered life threatening, and should therefore be treated conservatively and as medical emergencies.

HEAD

SECTION II

Temporomandibular

Chvostek Test

TEST POSITIONING:
The subject can either sit or stand.

ACTION:
The examiner taps over the masseter muscle and parotid gland (Figure 4).

POSITIVE FINDING:
Twitching of the facial muscles, especially the masseter, is indicative of positive findings for facial nerve pathology.

SPECIAL CONSIDERATIONS/COMMENTS:
Twitching of the facial muscles may also be a result of low calcium levels in the blood.

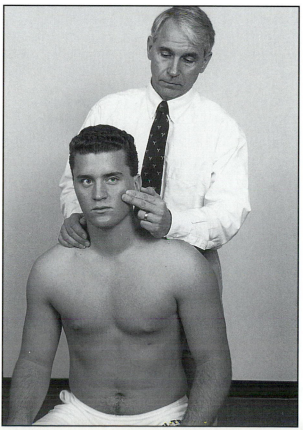

FIGURE 4

Loading Test

TEMPOROMANDIBULAR

TEST POSITIONING:
The subject is seated upright in a chair.

ACTION:
The examiner places a cotton roll between the molars on the uninvolved side and instructs the subject to bite down forcefully.

POSITIVE FINDING:
The reporting of pain by the subject indicates a positive finding, which may be reflective of an anteriorly dislocated disc.

SPECIAL CONSIDERATIONS/COMMENTS:
The subject may be instructed to chew on the cotton as opposed to forcefully biting down. A positive finding for pain may suggest any number of temporomandibular pathologies.

Palpation Test

TEST POSITIONING:
The subject is seated upright in a chair.

ACTION:
The examiner faces the subject and places his little fingers in the subject's ears. The subject is instructed to repeatedly open and close the mouth while the examiner applies pressure in an anterior direction using the pads of the little fingers (Figures 6A and 6B).

POSITIVE FINDING:
The subject's reporting of pain or discomfort during the opening and closing of the mouth when pressure is applied indicates a positive test. This may be a result of inflammation to the synovium of the joint.

SPECIAL CONSIDERATIONS/COMMENTS:
The subjective reporting of pain can be a result of any pathology to the temporomandibular joint.

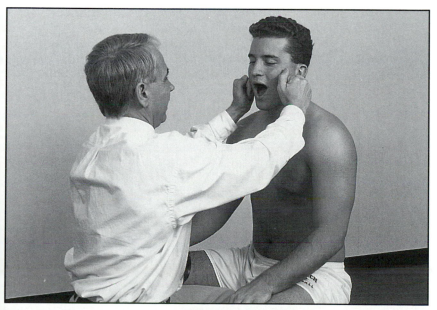

FIGURE 6A

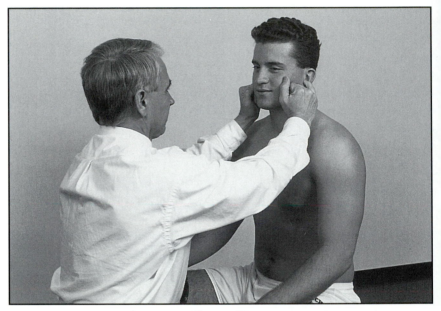

FIGURE 6B

SECTION III

Cervical Spine

Foraminal Compression Test (Spurling)

TEST POSITIONING:
With subject seated comfortably, the examiner rests the volar surface of both hands on the top of the subject's head (Figure 7A).

ACTION:
The examiner applies a downward pressure while the subject laterally flexes the head. The test is repeated with the subject laterally flexing to the opposite side (Figure 7B).

POSITIVE FINDING:
During the application of compression, a reporting of pain into the upper extremity toward the same side that the head is laterally flexed is positive. This indicates pressure on a nerve root which can be correlated by the dermatomal distribution of the pain.

SPECIAL CONSIDERATIONS/COMMENTS:
Precautions (and possibly avoidance) should be taken with compression of the vertebral area with a subject who has been diagnosed with conditions such as osteoarthritis, rheumatoid arthritis, osteoporosis, and spinal stenosis.

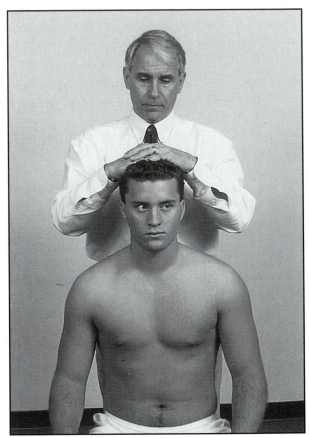

FIGURE 7A

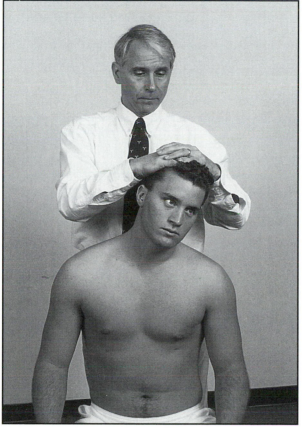

FIGURE 7B

Foraminal Distraction Test

TEST POSITIONING:
With the subject seated, the examiner places one hand under the subject's chin and the other hand around the occiput (Figure 8).

ACTION:
The examiner slowly distracts the subject's head from the trunk.

POSITIVE FINDING:
The finding is positive when existing complaints of pain decrease or disappear during the distraction. This indicates that a nerve root compression may exist while the subject sustains normal posture and/or positioning.

SPECIAL CONSIDERATIONS/COMMENTS:
Distraction of the cervical area for the assessment of a nerve root impingement should not be performed on a subject who has vertebral instability.

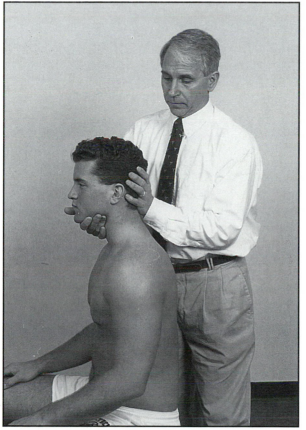

FIGURE 8

Vertebral Artery Test

TEST POSITIONING:
The subject is supine, and the examiner is seated with hands supporting the subject's head.

ACTION:
Slowly extend, rotate, and laterally flex the subject's cervical spine to each side. Then observe the subject for dizziness, blurred vision, nystagmus, slurred speech, or loss of consciousness (Figure 9).

POSITIVE FINDING:
Dizziness, blurred vision, nystagmus, slurred speech, or loss of consciousness are indicative of partial or complete occlusion of the vertebral artery.

SPECIAL CONSIDERATIONS/COMMENTS:
The aforementioned signs and symptoms should be considered contraindications for such treatments as traction and joint mobilizations.

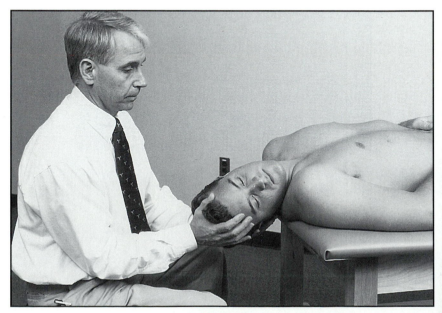

FIGURE 9

Valsalva Maneuver

TEST POSITIONING:
The subject should be seated. The examiner stands next to the subject.

ACTION:
The examiner asks the subject to take a deep breath and hold while bearing down as if having a bowel movement.

POSITIVE FINDING:
Increased pain due to increased intrathecal pressure, which may be secondary to a space-occupying lesion, herniated disk, tumor, or osteophyte in the cervical canal is positive. Pain may be localized or referred to corresponding dermatome.

SPECIAL CONSIDERATIONS/COMMENTS:
The increased pressure may alter venous function and cause dizziness or unconsciousness. The examiner should be prepared to steady the subject.

Swallowing Test

TEST POSITIONING:
The subject should be seated. The examiner stands next to the subject.

ACTION:
The examiner asks the subject to swallow.

POSITIVE FINDING:
Increased pain or difficulty swallowing (dysphagia) caused by anterior cervical spine obstructions such as vertebral subluxations, osteophyte protrusion, soft tissue swelling, or tumors in the anterior cervical spine region is positive.

SPECIAL CONSIDERATIONS/COMMENTS:
Be certain the subject's head is neutral, as swallowing becomes more difficult with the neck extended.

Empty Can (Supraspinatus) Test

TEST POSITIONING:
The subject stands with both shoulders abducted to 90 degrees, horizontally adducted 30 degrees, and internally rotated so the subject's thumbs face the floor (Figure 12).

ACTION:
The examiner resists the subject's attempts to actively abduct both shoulders.

POSITIVE FINDING:
Involvement of the supraspinatus muscle and/or tendon is suspected with noted weakness and/or a report of pain.

SPECIAL CONSIDERATIONS/COMMENTS:
Weakness of the supraspinatus muscle may be a result of suprascapular nerve involvement. Reported pain my be indicative of tendonitis and/or impingement.

SHOULDER

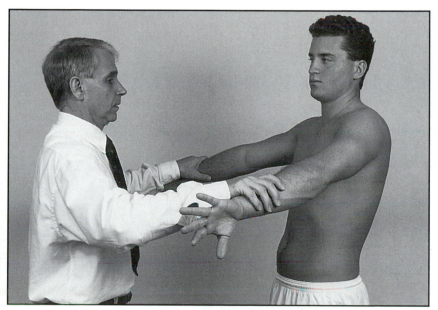

FIGURE 12

Yergason Test

TEST POSITIONING:
The subject is seated with the elbow flexed to 90 degrees and stabilized against the thorax, and the forearm in a pronated position. The examiner places one hand along the subject's forearm and the other hand on the upper portion of the subject's humerus, near the bicipital groove (Figure 13A).

ACTION:
The examiner resists the subject's attempt to supinate the forearm and externally rotate the humerus (Figure 13B).

POSITIVE FINDING:
Pain that is reported to exist in the area of the bicipital groove is a positive finding that may indicate bicipital tendinitis.

SPECIAL CONSIDERATIONS/COMMENTS:
This is a difficult test to perform. One may be just as accurate to assess bicipital tendinitis by simply palpating the long head of the biceps tendon in its bicipital groove.

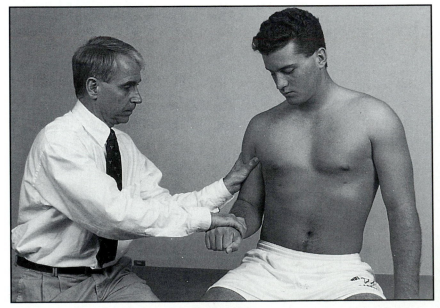

FIGURE 13A

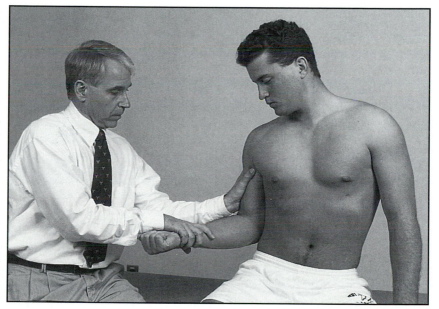

FIGURE 13B

Speed's Test

TEST POSITIONING:
The subject is seated on a table or standing with the involved shoulder flexed to 90 degrees, the elbow fully extended, and the forearm supinated. The examiner places one hand along the volar aspect of the subject's forearm and the other hand on the proximal aspect of the subject's humerus near the area of the bicipital groove (Figure 14).

ACTION:
The examiner resists the subject's attempt to actively forward flex the humerus.

POSITIVE FINDING:
Tenderness and/or pain in the bicipital groove is a positive finding that may suggest bicipital tendinitis.

SPECIAL CONSIDERATIONS/COMMENTS:
The examiner should carefully watch that the forearm is supinated and that the subject does not use accessory muscles to mask any existing weakness.

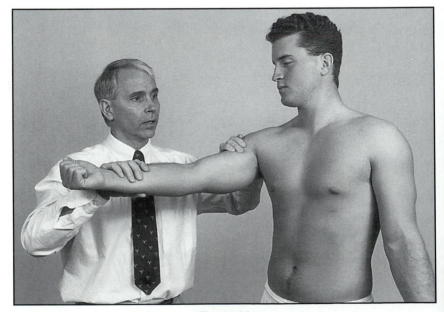

FIGURE 14

Drop Arm Test

TEST POSITIONING:
The subject is seated on a table or standing.

ACTION:
The examiner passively abducts the subject's involved arm to 90
degrees and then instructs the subject to slowly lower the arm to the
side (Figures 15A and 15B).

POSITIVE FINDING:
The subject is unable to slowly return the arm to the side and/or has
significant pain when attempting to perform the task. This is indicative
of rotator cuff pathology.

SPECIAL CONSIDERATIONS/COMMENTS:
If the examiner suspects rotator cuff pathology prior to performing the
test, he should prepare to rapidly comfort the subject in the event that
the subject does experience an inability to control the adduction movement of the arm.

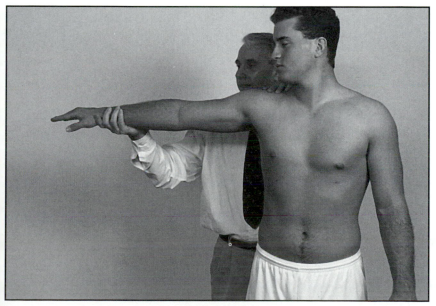

FIGURE 15A

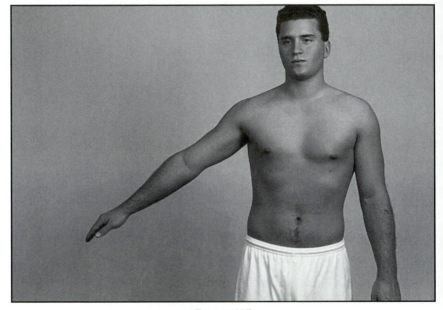

FIGURE 15B

Apley's Scratch Test

TEST POSITIONING:
The subject may be seated or standing. The examiner stands next to the subject.

ACTION:
1. The subject is instructed to take one hand and touch the opposite shoulder. Repeat with other hand to opposite side (Figure 16A).

POSITIVE FINDING:
1. Asymmetrical results from side to side are positive. The inability to touch the opposite shoulder is indicative of limited glenohumeral adduction, internal rotation, and horizontal flexion. Limits in scapular protraction may also produce asymmetrical results.

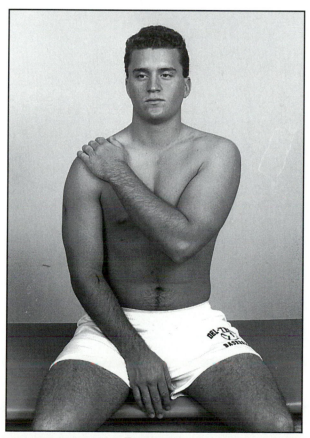

FIGURE 16A

ACTION:
2. The subject is then instructed to place the arm overhead and reach behind the neck as if scratching the upper back. Repeat with opposite side (Figure 16B).

POSITIVE FINDING:
2. Asymmetrical results from side to side are positive. Decreased motion on one side is indicative of limited glenohumeral abduction and external rotation, and scapular upward rotation and elevation.

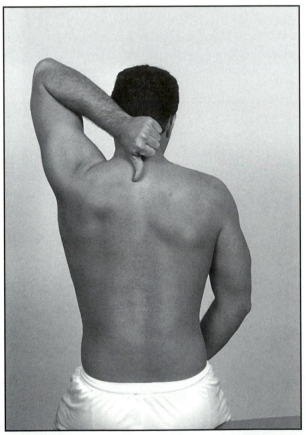

FIGURE 16B

ACTION:
3. The subject is then instructed to place the hand in the small of the back and reach upward as far as possible. Repeat with opposite side (Figure 16C).

POSITIVE FINDING:
3. Asymmetrical results from side to side are positive. Decreased motion on one side is indicative of limited glenohumeral adduction and internal rotation, and scapular retraction and downward rotation.

SPECIAL CONSIDERATIONS/COMMENTS:
Each of these movements is an active test of the functional mobility of the shoulder. Care should be taken to isolate movements that are restricted. It is not uncommon for a subject to have slightly greater restriction on the dominant shoulder as compared to the non-dominant shoulder, due to increased muscle mass on the dominant side.

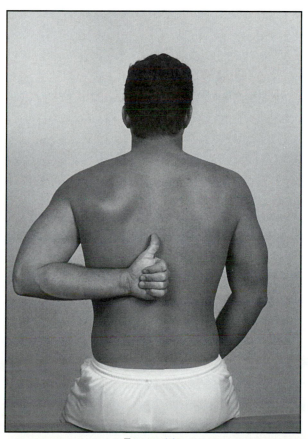

FIGURE 16C

Cross-Over Impingement Test

TEST POSITIONING:
The subject is seated. The examiner is standing with one hand on the posterior aspect of the subject's shoulder to stabilize the trunk and the other hand grasping the subject's elbow on the test arm.

ACTION:
With the subject's trunk stabilized, maximally horizontally adduct the test shoulder (Figure 17).

POSITIVE FINDING:
Superior shoulder pain is indicative of acromioclavicular joint pathology. Anterior shoulder pain is indicative of subscapularis, supraspinatus, and/or biceps long head pathology. Posterior shoulder pain is indicative of infraspinatus, teres minor, and/or posterior capsule pathology.

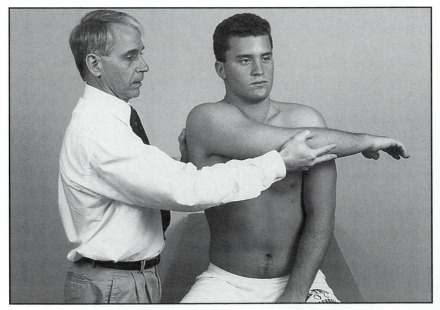

FIGURE 17

Neer Impingement Test

TEST POSITIONING:
The subject is sitting or standing with both upper extremities relaxed. The examiner is standing with one hand on the scapula (posteriorly) and the other hand grasping the subject's elbow (anteriorly).

ACTION:
With the subject's scapula stabilized, maximally forward flex the test shoulder (Figure 18).

POSITIVE FINDING:
Shoulder pain and apprehension are indicative of shoulder impingement, particularly of the supraspinatus and biceps long head tendons.

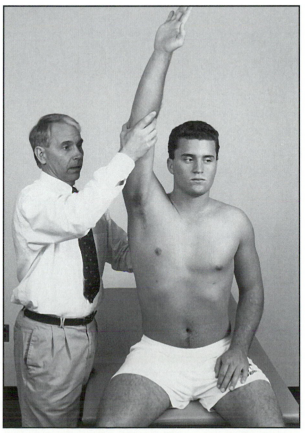

FIGURE 18

Hawkins-Kennedy Impingement Test

TEST POSITIONING:
The subject is sitting or standing with both upper extremities relaxed. The examiner is standing with one hand grasping the subject's elbow and the other hand grasping the subject's wrist, both on the test arm.

ACTION:
The examiner forward flexes the shoulder to 90 degrees and then internally rotates the subject's test shoulder (Figure 19).

POSITIVE FINDING:
Shoulder pain and apprehension are indicative of shoulder impingement, particularly of the supraspinatus tendon.

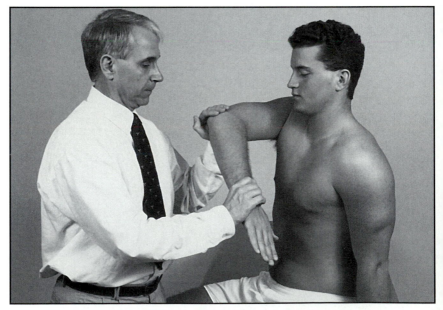

FIGURE 19

Sternoclavicular (SC) Joint Stress Test

TEST POSITIONING:
The subject is seated with the involved arm relaxed at the side. The examiner stands in front of the subject placing one hand on the proximal end of the subject's clavicle and the other hand on the spine of the scapula (Figure 20).

ACTION:
The examiner applies gentle downward and inward pressure on the clavicle, noting any movement at the SC joint.

POSITIVE FINDING:
Pain and/or movement of the clavicle indicates a sternoclavicular ligament sprain, possibly involving the costoclavicular ligament.

SPECIAL CONSIDERATIONS/COMMENTS:
This test should not be performed if there is obvious SC joint deformity.

SHOULDER

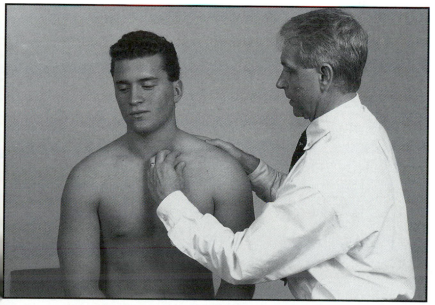

FIGURE 20

Acromioclavicular (AC) Joint Distraction Test

TEST POSITIONING:
The subject is seated with the involved arm relaxed at the side and the elbow flexed to 90 degrees. The examiner stands on the involved side holding the subject's arm just above the elbow crease. The examiner's other hand is placed over the involved AC joint (Figure 21).

ACTION:
The examiner applies gentle downward pressure on the arm, noting any movement at the AC joint.

POSITIVE FINDING:
Pain and/or movement of the scapula inferior to the clavicle is positive, indicating acromioclavicular and coracoclavicular ligament sprains.

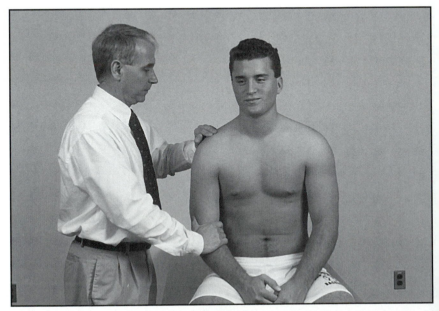

FIGURE 21

Acromioclavicular (AC) Joint Compression Test

TEST POSITIONING:
The subject is seated with the involved arm relaxed at the side. The examiner stands on the involved side, placing one hand on the subject's clavicle and the other hand on the spine of the scapula (Figure 22).

ACTION:
The examiner gently squeezes the hands together, noting any movement at the AC joint.

POSITIVE FINDING:
Pain and/or movement of the clavicle is positive, indicating an acromioclavicular and/or coracoclavicular ligament sprain.

SPECIAL CONSIDERATIONS/COMMENTS:
This test should not be performed if there is obvious AC joint deformity.

SHOULDER

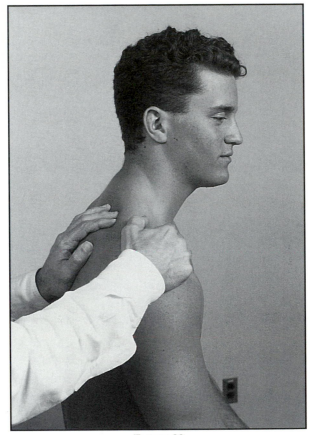

FIGURE 22

Piano Key Sign

TEST POSITIONING:
The subject is seated on a table or standing facing the examiner.

ACTION:
The examiner applies pressure to the subject's distal clavicle in an inferior direction (Figure 23A).

POSITIVE FINDING:
The examiner is able to use inferior pressure to depress the clavicle into its normal resting position and subsequently watch the clavicle elevate again once the pressure is removed (Figure 23B). This finding is indicative of the instability of the acromioclavicular joint on the involved side.

SPECIAL CONSIDERATIONS/COMMENTS:
The examiner should always use a bilateral comparison when assessing the range of elevation and depression of the involved clavicle. Significant clavicular elevation may also indicate coracoclavicular joint involvement.

SHOULDER

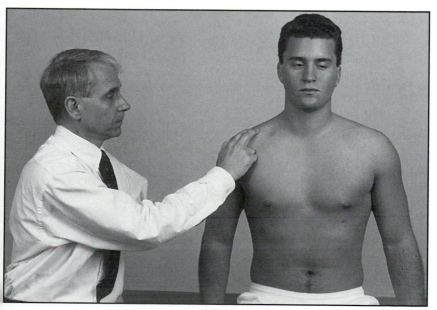

FIGURE 23A

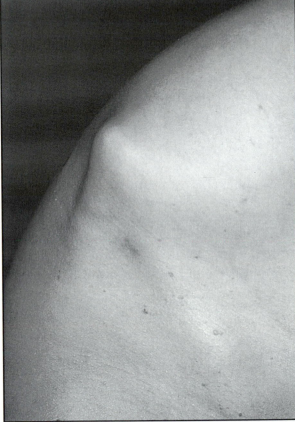

FIGURE 23B

Apprehension Test (Anterior)

TEST POSITIONING:
The subject lies supine on a table.

ACTION:
With the subject's involved shoulder in 90 degrees of abduction, the examiner slowly externally rotates the shoulder (Figure 24).

POSITIVE FINDING:
This test can be interpreted as a positive finding when the subject either looks or expresses feelings of apprehension toward further movement in the externally rotated direction. This test is used to mimic the positioning and movement of an anterior dislocation of the glenohumeral joint, thus recreating a subject's episode of instability.

SPECIAL CONSIDERATIONS/COMMENTS:
Simple indicating or reporting of apprehension to a movement does not necessarily indicate a dislocation of the glenohumeral joint.

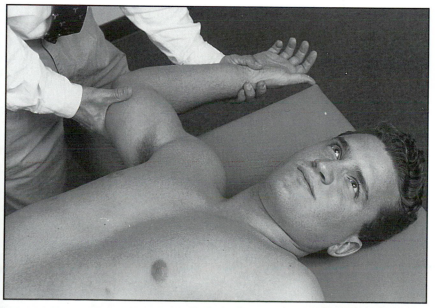

FIGURE 24

Apprehension Test (Posterior)

TEST POSITIONING:
The subject lies supine on a table. The examiner grasps the subject's elbow with one hand and stabilizes the ipsilateral and involved shoulder with the other hand.

ACTION:
The examiner places the subject's involved shoulder in a position of 90 degrees of flexion and internal rotation, while applying a posterior force through the long axis of the humerus (Figure 25).

POSITIVE FINDING:
This test can be interpreted as a positive finding when the subject either looks or expresses feelings of apprehension toward further movement in the posterior direction. This test is used to mimic the positioning and movement of a posterior dislocation of the glenohumeral joint, thus recreating a subject's episode of instability.

SPECIAL CONSIDERATIONS/COMMENTS:
Simple indicating or reporting of apprehension to a movement does not necessarily indicate a dislocation of the glenohumeral joint.

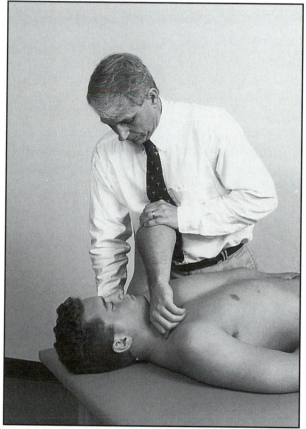

FIGURE 25

Sulcus Sign

TEST POSITIONING:
The subject is seated with the forearms and hands resting in the lap, and the examiner is standing with the proximal hand grasping the subject's scapula (superiorly) and the distal hand grasping the subject's elbow (Figure 26).

ACTION:
With the scapula stabilized, apply an inferior (distraction) force with the distal hand.

POSITIVE FINDING:
Excessive inferior humeral translation with a visible and/or palpable "step-off" or "sulcus" deformity immediately inferior to the acromion (laterally) is indicative of multi-directional instability.

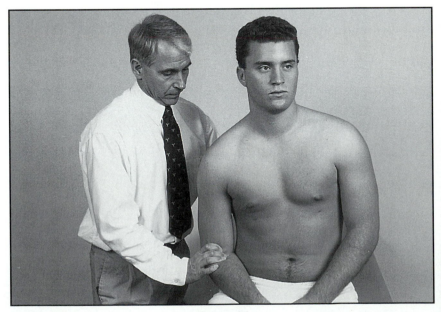

FIGURE 26

Anterior Drawer Test

TEST POSITIONING:
The subject is lying supine with the glenohumeral joint positioned at the edge of the table. The examiner stands next to the involved shoulder, placing one hand around the humerus below the surgical neck. The other hand stabilizes the scapula by placing the fingers behind the subject on the spine of the scapula and the thumb over the coracoid process (Figure 27).

ACTION:
The subject must remain relaxed while the examiner passively abducts the glenohumeral joint 70 to 80 degrees, forward flexes 0 to 10 degrees, and externally rotates 0 to 10 degrees. While stabilizing the scapula, the examiner firmly glides the head of the humerus anteriorly while applying slight distraction to the glenohumeral joint.

POSITIVE FINDING:
Increased anterior translation of the humeral head relative to the scapula/glenoid fossa may be indicative of anterior instability. The patient may exhibit apprehension if the test is positive.

SHOULDER

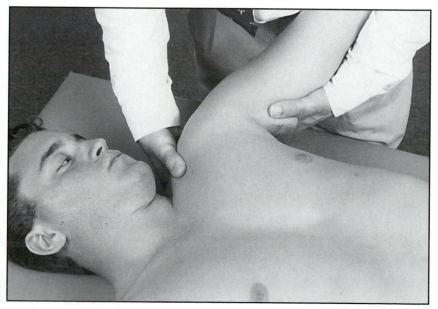

FIGURE 27

Posterior Drawer Test

TEST POSITIONING:
The subject is lying supine. The examiner stands next to the involved shoulder, grabs the subject's arm at the elbow, passively abducts the shoulder to 90 degrees, and horizontally flexes the shoulder 20 to 30 degrees. The subject's elbow is flexed in a relaxed position. The examiner stabilizes the scapula by placing the other hand posterior to the shoulder joint capsule with the thumb over the coracoid process (Figure 28A).

ACTION:
While stabilizing the scapula, the examiner internally rotates the humerus and applies downward pressure, pushing the humeral head posteriorly. The examiner notes any posterior movement of the head (Figure 28B).

POSITIVE FINDING:
Increased posterior instability of the humeral head relative to the scapula/glenoid fossa may be indicative of posterior instability. The subject may exhibit apprehension if the test is positive.

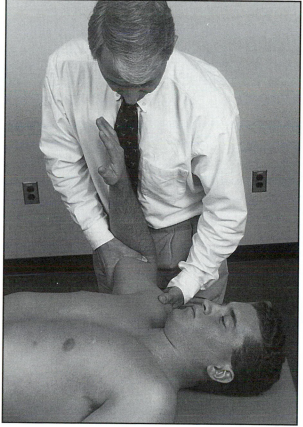

FIGURE 28A

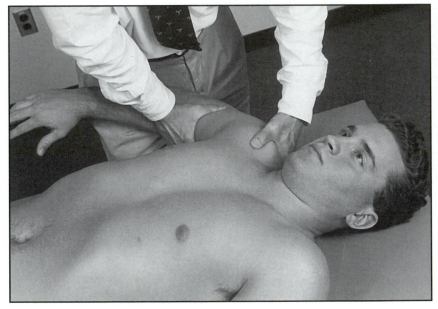

FIGURE 28B

Jobe Relocation Test

TEST POSITIONING:
The subject is supine with the test shoulder in 90 degrees of abduction and full external rotation. The examiner is standing with the distal hand grasping the subject's wrist and hand, and the proximal hand over the subject's humeral head (anteriorly) (Figure 29).

ACTION:
Apply a posterior force to the humeral head.

POSITIVE FINDING:
A reduction of pain and apprehension and commonly an increase in shoulder external rotation are indicative of anterior instability.

SPECIAL CONSIDERATIONS/COMMENTS:
This test should be performed immediately following the Apprehension Test.

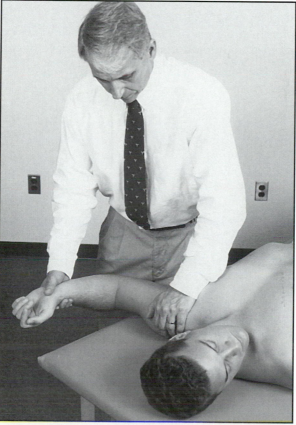

FIGURE 29

Grind Test

TEST POSITIONING:
The subject lies supine on a table with the shoulder abducted to 90 degrees and the elbow flexed to 90 degrees on the involved side. The examiner grasps the subject's elbow with one hand and the subject's proximal humerus with the other hand (Figure 30).

ACTION:
The examiner applies compression to the glenoid labrum while attempting to rotate the humeral head 360 degrees around the surface of the glenoid fossa.

POSITIVE FINDING:
A positive finding of a grinding or clunking sensation may be indicative of a glenoid labrum tear to the specific location which is being compressed.

SPECIAL CONSIDERATIONS/COMMENTS:
This test should be done carefully since the application of excessive pressure combined with rotation may further damage the glenoid labrum.

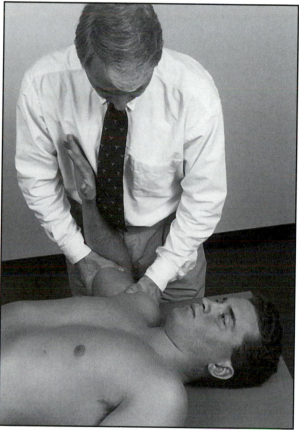

FIGURE 30

Clunk Test

TEST POSITIONING:
The subject lies supine on a table. The examiner places one hand on the posterior aspect of the subject's humeral head, and the other hand proximal to the subject's elbow joint along the distal humerus (Figure 31A).

ACTION:
The examiner passively abducts and externally rotates the subject's arm overhead and applies an anterior force to the humerus. (The examiner may also choose to internally rotate the humerus at the same time the anterior force is being applied). The examiner then circumducts the humeral head about the glenoid labrum (Figure 31B).

POSITIVE FINDING:
A positive finding of a grinding or clunking sensation may be indicative of a glenoid labrum tear.

SPECIAL CONSIDERATIONS/COMMENTS:
The subject may appear to have a positive test or even show apprehension in this position, if an underlying anterior and/or inferior instability of the glenohumeral joint exists.

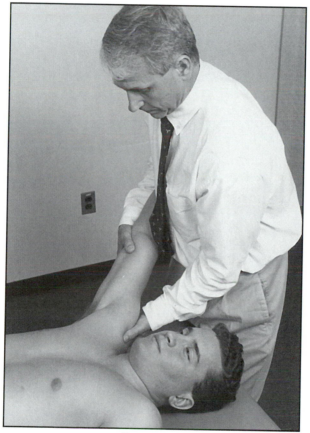

FIGURE 31A

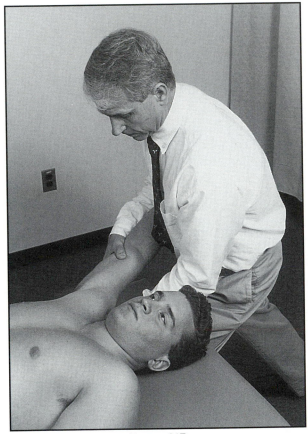

FIGURE 31B

O'Brien Test

TEST POSITIONING:
The subject is sitting or standing with the test shoulder in 90 degrees of forward flexion, 30 to 45 degrees of horizontal adduction and maximal internal rotation. The examiner is standing with one hand grasping the subject's test wrist (medially) (Figure 32A).

ACTION:
The subject horizontally adducts and flexes the test shoulder against the examiner's manual resistance (Figure 32B).

POSITIVE FINDING:
Pain and/or popping are indicative of a superior labrum anterior-posterior (SLAP) lesion.

SPECIAL CONSIDERATIONS/COMMENTS:
The O'Brien Test is considered to be the most accurate test for assessing SLAP lesions; however, the sensitivity of this and other SLAP lesion tests is questionable.

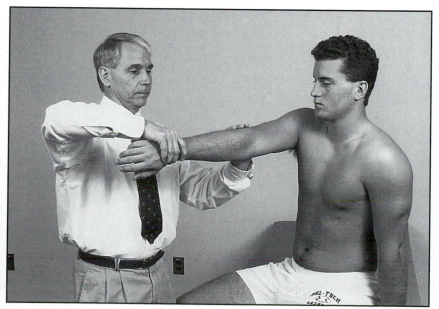

FIGURE 32A

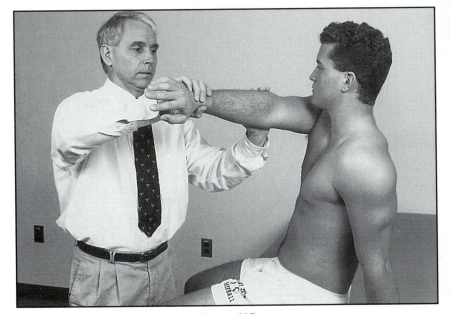

FIGURE 32B

Brachial Plexus Stretch Test

TEST POSITIONING:
The subject is seated. The examiner stands behind the subject and places one hand on the side of the subject's head and the other hand on the shoulder of the same side.

ACTION:
The examiner laterally flexes the subject's head while applying gentle downward pressure on the shoulder (Figure 33).

POSITIVE FINDING:
Pain that radiates into the subject's arm that is opposite to the laterally flexed neck indicates a positive finding.

SPECIAL CONSIDERATIONS/COMMENTS:
If pain is in the neck on the side toward lateral flexion, a pinched nerve or facet joint impingement may exist. This test should not be performed if a cervical fracture or dislocation is suspected.

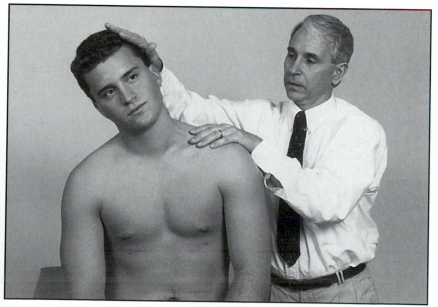

FIGURE 33

Adson Maneuver

TEST POSITIONING:
The subject is sitting or standing, and the examiner is standing with fingers over the radial artery (distally) (Figure 34A).

ACTION:
Externally rotate and extend the subject's test arm while palpating the radial pulse. The subject then extends and rotates the neck toward the test arm and takes a deep breath (Figure 34B).

POSITIVE FINDING:
A diminished or absent radial pulse is indicative of Thoracic Outlet Syndrome, secondary to compression of the subclavian artery by the scalene muscles.

SPECIAL CONSIDERATIONS/COMMENTS:
This test assesses vascular structures only, and has a high incidence (>50%) of false positive findings.

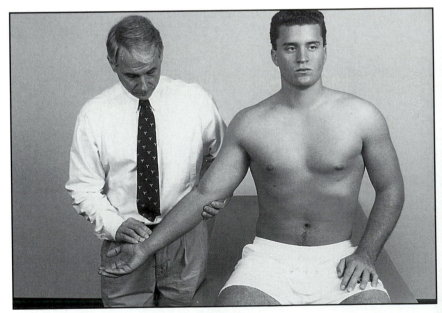

FIGURE 34A

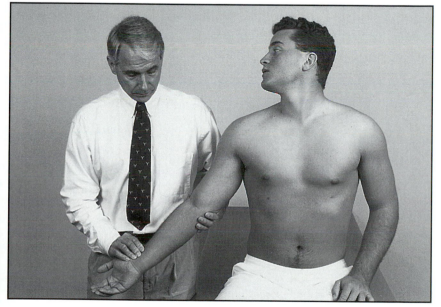

FIGURE 34B

Allen Test

TEST POSITIONING:
The subject is seated or standing with the test shoulder in 90 degrees of abduction and external rotation, and the elbow in 90 degrees of flexion. The examiner is standing with fingers over the radial artery (distally).

ACTION:
The subject rotates the neck away from the test arm while the examiner palpates the radial pulse (Figure 35).

POSITIVE FINDING:
A diminished or absent radial pulse is indicative of Thoracic Outlet Syndrome.

SPECIAL CONSIDERATIONS/COMMENTS:
This test assesses vascular structures only, and has a high incidence (>50%) of false positive findings.

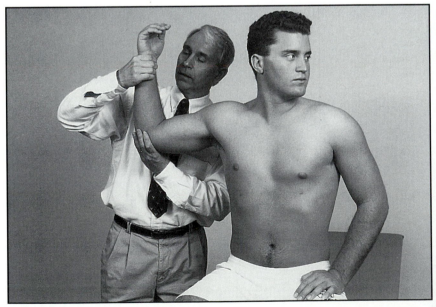

FIGURE 35

Roo Test

Test Positioning:
The subject is sitting or standing with both shoulders in 90 degrees of abduction and external rotation, and the elbows in 90 degrees of flexion.

Action:
The subject rapidly opens and closes both hands for 3 minutes (Figures 36A and 36B).

Positive Finding:
The inability to maintain the test position, diminished motor function of the hands, and/or loss of sensation in the upper extremities are indicative of Thoracic Outlet Syndrome, secondary to neurovascular compromise.

Special Considerations/Comments:
This test evaluates both neural and vascular structures and is considered to be the most accurate clinical test for assessing Thoracic Outlet Syndrome.

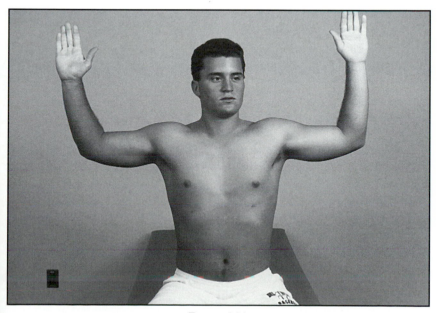

Figure 36A

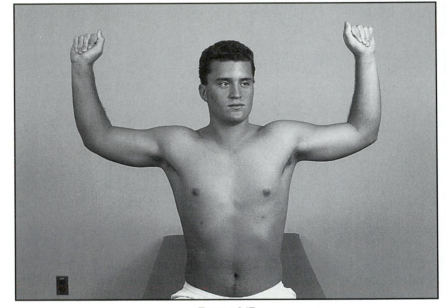

FIGURE 36B

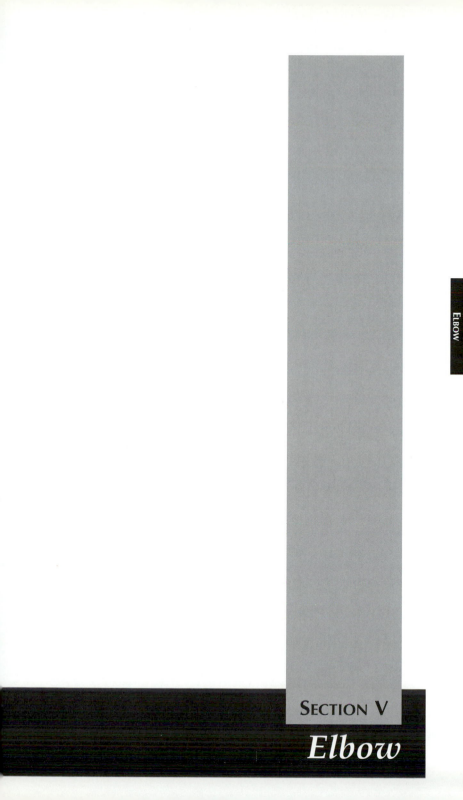

SECTION V

Elbow

Resistive Tennis Elbow Test (Cozen's Test)

TEST POSITIONING:
The subject is seated. The examiner stabilizes the involved elbow while palpating along the lateral epicondyle (Figure 37A).

ACTION:
With a closed fist, the subject pronates and radially deviates the forearm, and extends the wrist against the examiner's resistance (Figure 37B).

POSITIVE FINDING:
A report of pain along the lateral epicondyle region of the humerus, or objective muscle weakness as a result of complaints of discomfort may indicate lateral epicondylitis.

ELBOW

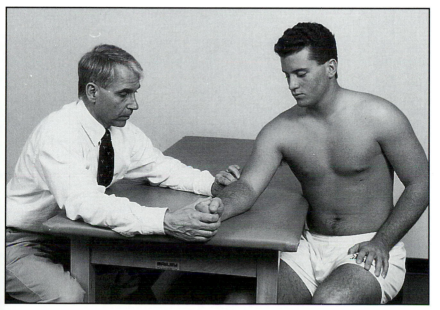

FIGURE 37A

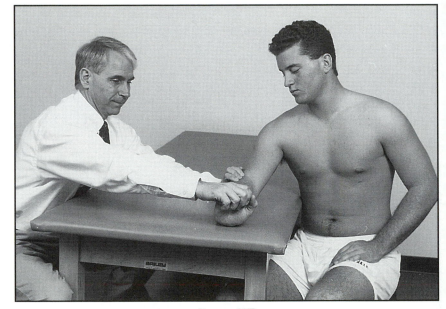

FIGURE 37B

Resistive Tennis Elbow Test

TEST POSITIONING:
The subject is seated. The examiner stabilizes the involved elbow with one hand and places the palm of the other hand on the dorsal aspect of the subject's hand just distal to the proximal interphalangeal joint of the third digit (Figure 38).

ACTION:
The subject extends the third digit against the examiner's resistance.

POSITIVE FINDING:
A reporting of pain along the lateral epicondyle region of the humerus, or objective muscle weakness as a result of complaints of discomfort may indicate lateral epicondylitis.

ELBOW

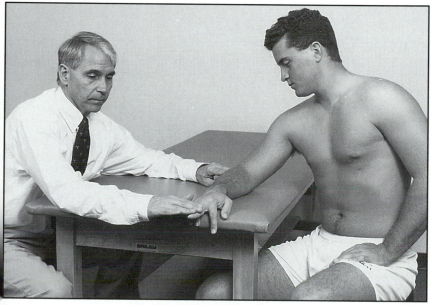

FIGURE 38

Passive Tennis Elbow Test

TEST POSITIONING:
The subject is seated with the involved elbow in full extension.

ACTION:
The examiner passively pronates the forearm and flexes the wrist of the subject (Figure 39A).

POSITIVE FINDING:
A reporting of pain along the lateral epicondyle region of the humerus may indicate lateral epicondylitis.

SPECIAL CONSIDERATIONS/COMMENTS:
The examiner may also palpate the involved lateral epicondyle region during the test to assess the tightness of the common extensor tendon origin. This test may also be performed with the elbow in flexion (Figure 39B).

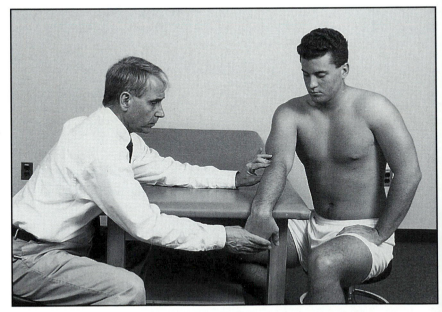

FIGURE 39A

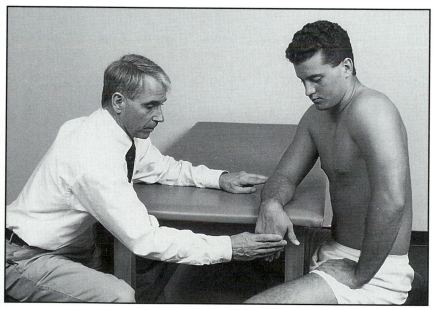

FIGURE 39B

Hyperextension Test

TEST POSITIONING:
The subject is seated or standing with the elbow fully extended and the forearm supinated. The examiner grasps the distal humerus at the areas of the medial and lateral epicondyles with one hand, while the other hand grasps the distal forearm of the subject (Figure 40).

ACTION:
The examiner passively extends the elbow until no further motion is available.

POSITIVE FINDING:
Elbow extension beyond 0 degrees is considered hyperextension. A positive finding of hyperextension may be attributed to a torn or stretched anterior capsule of the elbow.

SPECIAL CONSIDERATIONS/COMMENTS:
Assessing this motion should always be done bilaterally to determine the normal range of motion for the individual subject. Hyperextension findings may vary depending on the type of end feel noted.

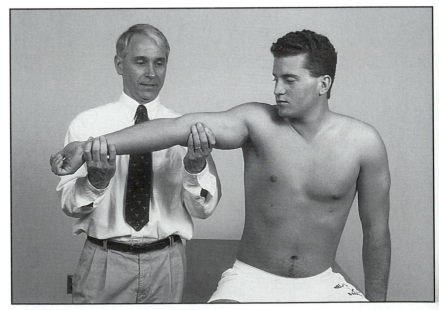

FIGURE 40

Elbow Flexion Test

TEST POSITIONING:
The subject may be seated or standing. The examiner stands next to the subject.

ACTION:
The subject is instructed to maximally flex the elbow and hold this position for 3 to 5 minutes (Figure 41).

POSITIVE FINDING:
Radiating pain into the median nerve distribution in the subject's arm and/or hand (ie, lateral forearm or tip of thumb, index and middle finger) is a positive finding. A positive test is indicative of cubital fossa syndrome.

SPECIAL CONSIDERATIONS/COMMENTS:
This test may also be indicative of ulnar nerve compromise in the ulnar groove if radiating pain extends into the subject's ulnar nerve distribution (ie, fourth and fifth digits).

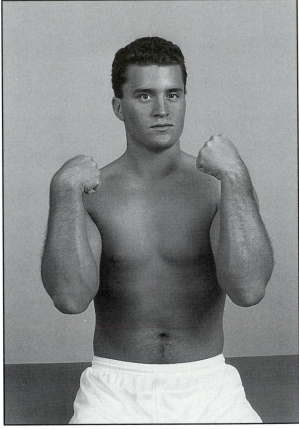

FIGURE 41

Varus Stress Test

TEST POSITIONING:
The subject is seated with the test elbow flexed to 20 to 30 degrees. The examiner is standing with the distal hand around subject's wrist (laterally) and the proximal hand over the subject's elbow joint (medially) (Figure 42).

ACTION:
With the wrist stabilized, apply a varus stress to the elbow with the proximal hand.

POSITIVE FINDING:
As compared to the uninvolved elbow, lateral elbow pain and/or increased varus movement with diminished or absent endpoint is indicative of damage to primarily the radial or lateral collateral ligament.

SPECIAL CONSIDERATIONS/COMMENTS:
The examiner must avoid allowing the humerus to internally or externally rotate during this test, as this will give the illusion of increased varus movement.

ELBOW

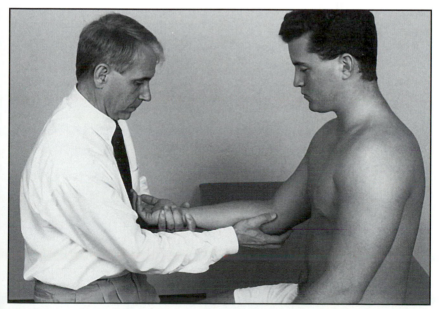

FIGURE 42

Valgus Stress Test

TEST POSITIONING:
The subject is seated with the test elbow flexed to 20 to 30 degrees. The examiner is standing with the distal hand around subject's wrist (medially) and the proximal hand over the subject's elbow joint (laterally) (Figure 43).

ACTION:
With the wrist stabilized, apply a valgus stress to the elbow with the proximal hand.

POSITIVE FINDING:
As compared to the uninvolved elbow, medial elbow pain and/or increased valgus movement with diminished or absent endpoint is indicative of damage to primarily the ulnar or medial collateral ligament.

SPECIAL CONSIDERATIONS/COMMENTS:
The examiner must avoid allowing the humerus to internally or externally rotate during this test, as this will give the illusion of increased valgus movement.

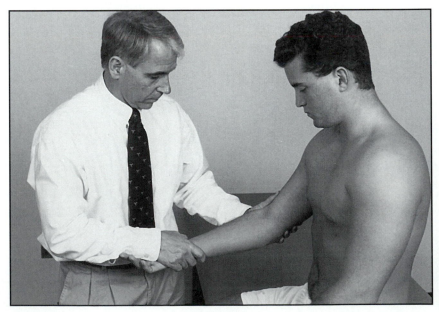

FIGURE 43

Tinel Sign

TEST POSITIONING:
The subject is seated with the elbow in slight flexion, and the examiner is standing with the distal hand grasping the subject's wrist (laterally).

ACTION:
With the wrist stabilized, tap the ulnar nerve in the ulnar notch (between the olecranon process and medial epicondyle) with the index finger (Figure 44).

POSITIVE FINDING:
Tingling along the ulnar distribution of the forearm, hand, and fingers is indicative of ulnar nerve compromise.

ELBOW

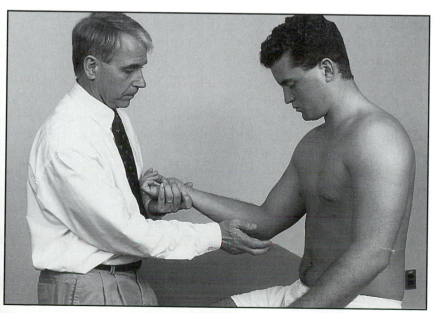

FIGURE 44

Pinch Grip Test

TEST POSITIONING:
The subject may be seated or standing. The examiner stands next to the subject.

ACTION:
The subject is instructed to pinch the tips of the thumb and index finger together (Figure 45).

POSITIVE FINDING:
The inability to touch the tips of the thumb and index finger together demonstrates a positive finding. Touching the pads of the thumb and index finger indicates pathology of the anterior interosseous nerve. There may be entrapment of the anterior interosseous nerve between the two heads of the pronator muscle.

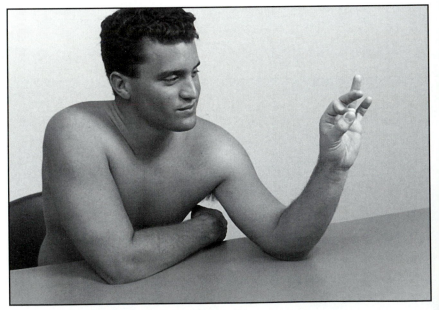

FIGURE 45

SECTION VI

Wrist & Hand

Tap or Percussion Test

TEST POSITIONING:
The subject may be seated or standing with the affected finger extended. The examiner stands in front of the subject.

ACTION:
The examiner applies a firm tap to the end of the finger being tested (Figures 46A and 46B). As an alternative method to tapping, the examiner may use a percussion hammer (Figure 46C).

POSITIVE FINDING:
Pain at the site of injury is indicative of a fracture. The vibration of tapping along the long axis of the bone will exaggerate pain at the fracture site.

SPECIAL CONSIDERATIONS/COMMENTS:
This test should not be performed if there is obvious deformity.

WRIST & HAND

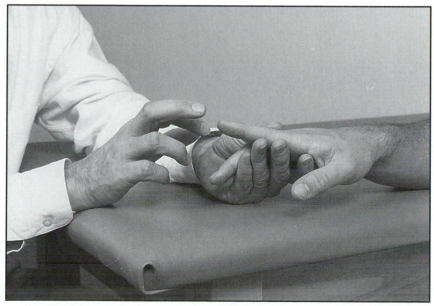

FIGURE 46A

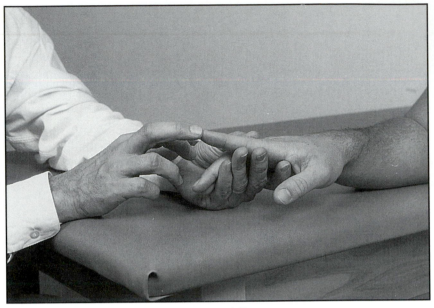

FIGURE 46B

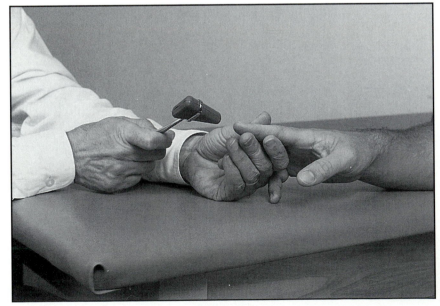

FIGURE 46C

Compression Test

TEST POSITIONING:
The subject may be seated or standing with the affected finger extended. The examiner stands in front of the subject.

ACTION:
The examiner holds the distal phalanx and applies compression along the long axis of the bone of the finger being tested (Figure 47).

POSITIVE FINDING:
Pain at the site of injury is indicative of a fracture.

SPECIAL CONSIDERATIONS/COMMENTS:
This test should not be performed if there is obvious deformity.

WRIST & HAND

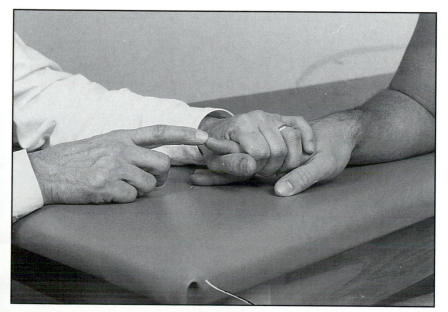

FIGURE 47

Long Finger Flexor Test

TEST POSITIONING:
The subject may be seated or standing.
1. The examiner stands in front of the subject holding the subject's fingers in extension except for the finger being tested (Figure 48A).
2. The examiner isolates the distal interphalangeal joint by stabilizing the metacarpophalangeal and proximal interphalangeal joints of the finger being tested (Figure 48B).

ACTION:
1. The subject is instructed to flex the finger being tested at the proximal interphalangeal joint.
2. The subject is instructed to flex the distal inter-phalangeal joint (Figure 48C).

POSITIVE FINDING:
If the subject is unable to flex the proximal interphalangeal joint, the flexor digitorum superficialis muscle is compromised. If the subject is unable to flex the distal interphalangeal, the flexor digitorum profundus muscle is compromised.

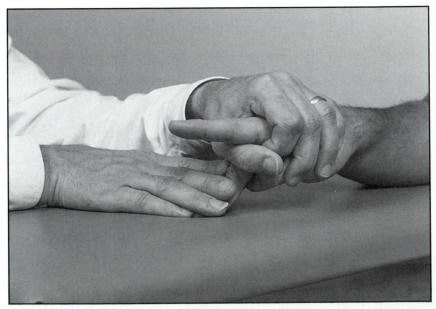

FIGURE 48A

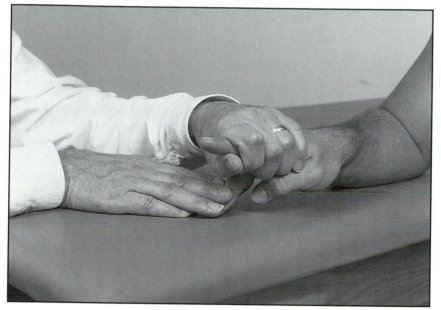

FIGURE 48B

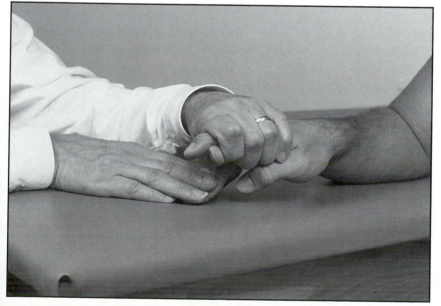

FIGURE 48C

Finkelstein Test

TEST POSITIONING:
The subject is sitting or standing and forms a fist around the thumb.
The examiner is standing with the proximal hand grasping the subject's forearm and the distal hand grasping the subject's fist, with the
subject's thumb in the examiner's thenar eminence.

ACTION:
While stabilizing the subject's forearm with the proximal hand, ulnarly
deviate the subject's wrist with the distal hand (Figure 49).

POSITIVE FINDING:
Pain over the abductor pollicis longus and extensor pollicis brevis ten-
dons, distally, is indicative of tenosynovitis in these tendons (de
Quervain's Disease).

SPECIAL CONSIDERATIONS/COMMENTS:
This test may create pain in uninvolved tissues.

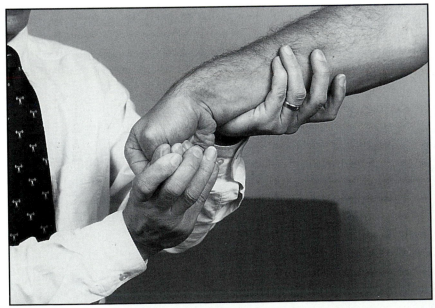

FIGURE 49

Phalen Test

TEST POSITIONING:
The subject is sitting or standing with the dorsal aspect of both hands in full contact, such that both wrists are maximally flexed (Figure 50).

ACTION:
A steady compressive force is applied through the subject's forearms such that the subject's wrists are maximally flexed for 1 minute.

POSITIVE FINDINGS:
Numbness and tingling in the median nerve distribution of the fingers (ie, thumb, index finger, middle finger, and lateral aspect of the ring finger) are indicative of Carpal Tunnel Syndrome, secondary to median nerve compression.

WRIST & HAND

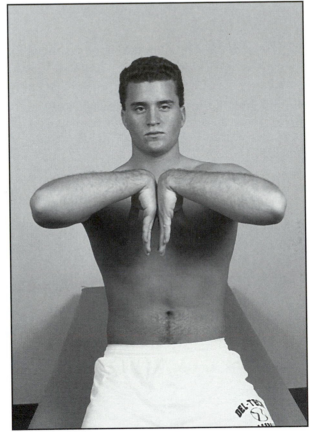

FIGURE 50

Tinel Test

TEST POSITIONING:
The subject is seated.

ACTION:
The examiner taps the volar aspect of the subject's wrist over the area of the carpal tunnel (Figures 51A and 51B).

POSITIVE FINDING:
Complaint's of tingling, paresthesia, or pain by the subject in the area of the thumb, index finger, middle finger, and radial one-half of the ring finger signal a positive test. This may be indicative of a compression of the median nerve in the carpal tunnel, or carpal tunnel syndrome.

SPECIAL CONSIDERATIONS/COMMENTS:
A positive tinel test at the wrist may appear if the median nerve is disrupted at any point of its path. Therefore, a positive finding should warrant the examiner to assess the integrity of the median nerve at the elbow, shoulder, and neck to rule out other pathology.

WRIST & HAND

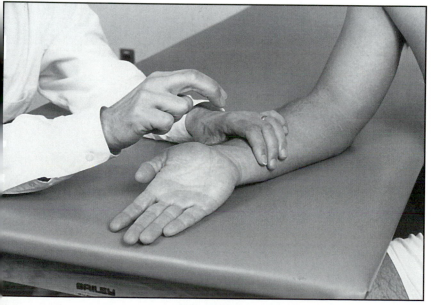

FIGURE 51A

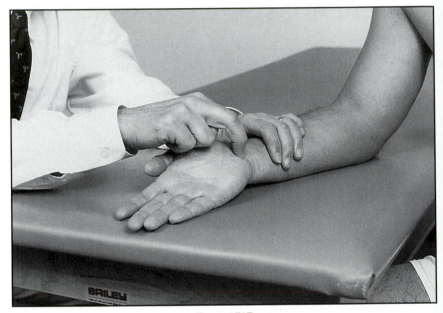

FIGURE 51B

Froment's Sign

TEST POSITIONING:
The subject may be seated or standing. The examiner is next to the subject.

ACTION:
The subject is instructed to hold a piece of paper between the thumb and index finger. The examiner then tries to pull the paper out (Figure 52).

POSITIVE FINDING:
Flexion of the subject's distal interphalangeal joint of the thumb is indicative of adductor pollicis muscle paralysis due to ulnar nerve damage.

SPECIAL CONSIDERATIONS/COMMENTS:
Simultaneous hyperextension of the metacarpophalangeal joint of the thumb is indicative of ulnar nerve compromise. This is known as Jeanne's sign.

WRIST & HAND

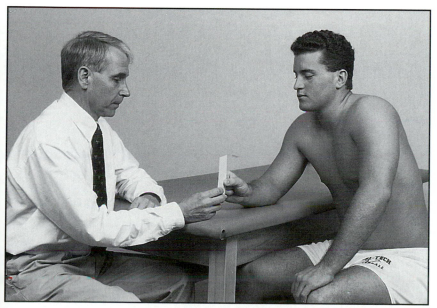

FIGURE 52

Wrinkle Test (Shrivel Test)

TEST POSITIONING:
The subject is seated.

ACTION:
The subject's fingers are placed in warm water for approximately 10 minutes (Figure 53). Upon removal, the examiner assesses the skin around the pulp area for any wrinkling.

POSITIVE FINDING:
A positive test is seen when the involved finger shows no signs of wrinkling, indicating denervated tissue.

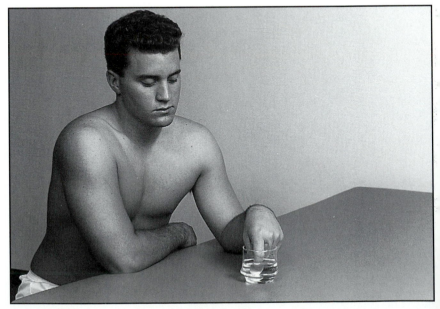

FIGURE 53

Digital Allen Test

TEST POSITIONING:
Both the subject and examiner are either seated or standing.

ACTION:
The subject is instructed to make a fist several times in succession in order to "pump" the blood out of the hand and fingers. The subject is then instructed to maintain a fist while the examiner compresses the radial artery with the thumb and the ulnar artery with the fingers (Figure 54A). As the subject relaxes the hand (Figure 54B), the examiner releases pressure from one artery at a time and observes the color of the hand and fingers (Figure 54C).

POSITIVE FINDING:
A delay in or absence of flushing of the radial or ulnar half of the hand and fingers is indicative of partial or complete occlusion of the radial or ulnar arteries, respectively.

WRIST & HAND

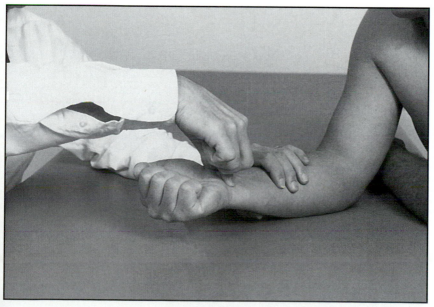

FIGURE 54A

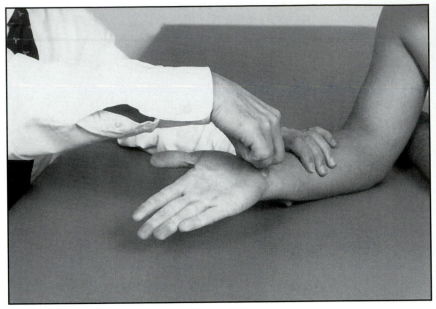

FIGURE 54B

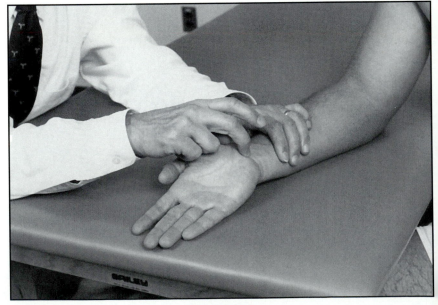

FIGURE 54C

Bunnel Littner Test

TEST POSITIONING:
The subject is seated with the metacarpophalangeal joint in slight extension.

ACTION:
The examiner passively flexes the proximal interphalangeal joint of the same ray and assesses the amount of flexion at the PIP (Figure 55A). The examiner then passively and slightly flexes the MCP, and again assesses the amount of flexion at the PIP (Figure 55B).

POSITIVE FINDING:
A positive finding is revealed if the PIP does not flex while the MCP is in an extended position. If the PIP does flex fully once the MCP is slightly flexed, intrinsic muscle tightness can be assumed. By contrast, if flexion of the PIP remains limited once the MCP is slightly flexed, capsular tightness can be assumed.

SPECIAL CONSIDERATIONS/COMMENTS:
Care should be taken by the examiner to retain extension and then flexion of the MCP joint while testing in each position to assess true PIP motion.

WRIST & HAND

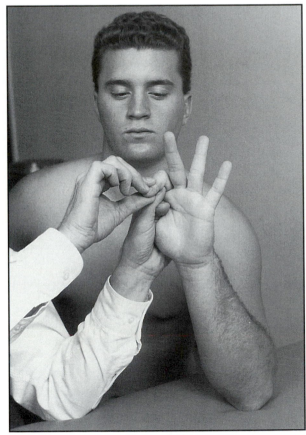

FIGURE 55A

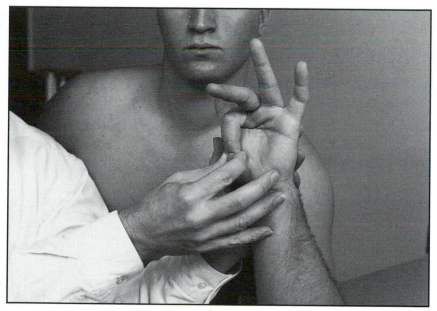

FIGURE 55B

Murphy's Sign

TEST POSITIONING:
The subject may be seated or standing. The examiner stands in front of the subject.

ACTION:
The subject is instructed to make a fist. The examiner notes the position of the third metacarpal (Figure 56).

POSITIVE FINDING:
If the subject's third metacarpal is level with the second and fourth metacarpal, a dislocated lunate is indicated.

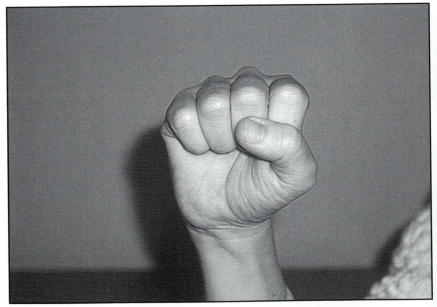

FIGURE 56

Watson Test

TEST POSITIONING:
The subject is seated. The examiner uses one hand to stabilize the distal forearm at the distal radial ulnar joint, while grasping the scaphoid bone of the subject with the other hand (Figure 57A).

ACTION:
The examiner mobilizes the scaphoid bone anteriorly and posteriorly while ulnarly and radially deviating the subject's wrist (Figure 57B).

POSITIVE FINDING:
Positive findings include a palpable subluxation and reduction of the scaphoid, and may be felt if an underlying carpal ligament tear is present.

SPECIAL CONSIDERATIONS/COMMENTS:
This test is easier to perform when the examiner grasps the scaphoid on the volar aspect with the thumb.

WRIST & HAND

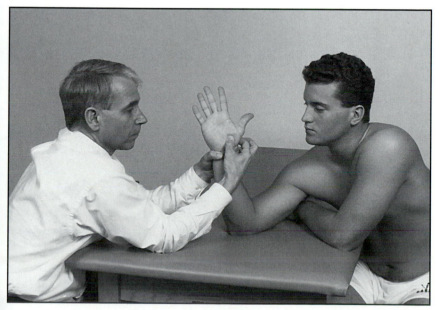

FIGURE 57A

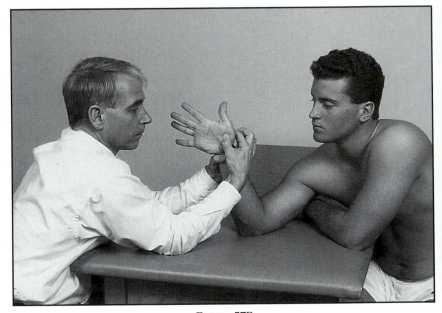

FIGURE 57B

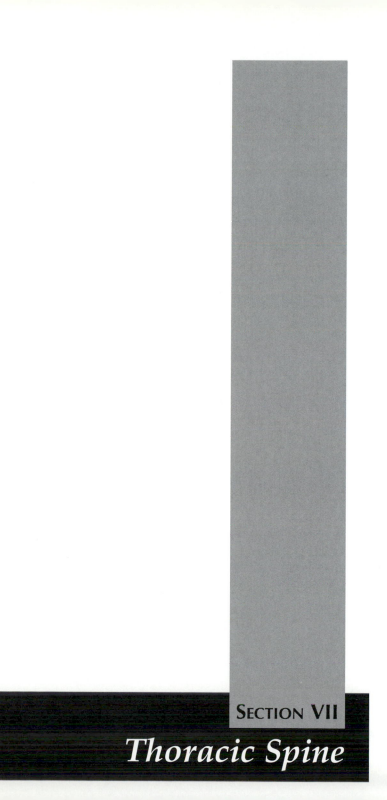

SECTION **VII**

Thoracic Spine

Kernig/Brudzinski Test

TEST POSITIONING:
The subject is lying supine with the hands cupped behind the head. The examiner stands next to the subject.

ACTION:
The subject is instructed to flex the cervical spine by lifting the head. Each hip is unilaterally flexed to no more than 90 degrees by the subject. The subject then flexes the knee to no more than 90 degrees. The opposite leg remains on the examining table (Figure 58).

POSITIVE FINDING:
The test is confirmed by increased pain, that either is localized or radiates into the lower extremity, with neck and hip flexion. The pain is relieved when the knee is flexed. The pain is indicative of meningeal irritation, nerve root impingement, or dural irritation that is exaggerated by elongating the spinal cord.

SPECIAL CONSIDERATIONS/COMMENTS:
The considerations are similar to the straight leg raise test except the neck is flexed and the hip is actively flexed. The neck flexion component of this test was developed by Kernig, whereas the hip flexion component was developed by Brudzinski.

THORACIC SPINE

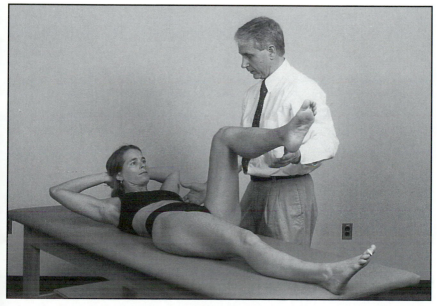

FIGURE 58

Lateral Rib Compression Test

TEST POSITIONING:
The subject is lying supine. The examiner stands next to the subject and places both hands on either side of the affected rib(s) (Figure 59).

ACTION:
The examiner compresses the lateral aspect of the rib cage bilaterally and then quickly releases.

POSITIVE FINDING:
Pain with compression or release of pressure indicates the possibility of a rib fracture, rib contusion, or costochondral separation.

SPECIAL CONSIDERATIONS/COMMENTS:
This test is contraindicated if there is an obvious deformity or possible lung trauma. Modification to this test is known as the Anterior/Posterior Rib Compression Test.

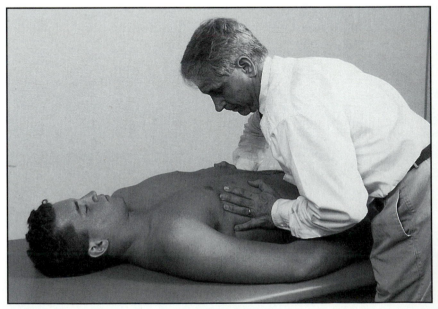

FIGURE 59

Anterior/Posterior Rib Compression Test

TEST POSITIONING:
The subject is lying supine. The examiner stands next to the subject and places one hand over the affected rib(s) and the other hand posterior to the rib cage (Figure 60).

ACTION:
The examiner compresses the rib cage anterior to posterior and quickly releases.

POSITIVE FINDING:
Pain with compression or release of pressure indicates the possibility of a rib fracture, rib contusion, or costochondral separation.

SPECIAL CONSIDERATIONS/COMMENTS:
This test is contraindicated if there is an obvious deformity or possible lung trauma. Modification to this test is known as the Lateral Rib Compression Test.

THORACIC SPINE

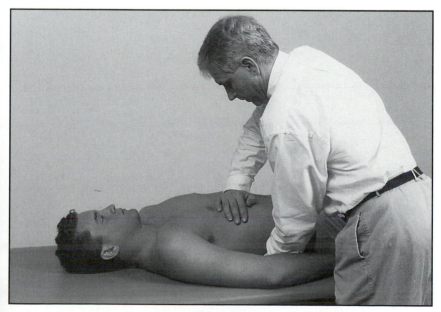

FIGURE 60

Inspiration/Expiration Breathing Test

TEST POSITIONING:
The subject is seated or standing. The examiner stands next to the subject.

ACTION:
The subject is instructed to breath in and out normally, then take in a deep breath followed by rapid expiration.

POSITIVE FINDING:
Normal breathing that is rapid and shallow is indicative of a rib fracture. Pain with deep inspiration may suggest a rib fracture, costochondral separation, or external intercostal muscle strain. Pain with forced expiration may indicate costochondral separation or internal intercostal muscle strain.

SPECIAL CONSIDERATIONS/COMMENTS:
With a rib fracture or costochondral separation, there is also pain with coughing, sneezing, and torso movement. Displaced rib fractures may jeopardize the function of the lungs and should be treated as a medical emergency.

SECTION VIII

Lumbar Spine

Valsalva Maneuver

TEST POSITIONING:
The subject should be seated. The examiner stands next to the subject.

ACTION:
The examiner asks the subject to take a deep breath and hold while bearing down as if having a bowel movement.

POSITIVE FINDING:
The test is confirmed by increased pain due to increased intrathecal pressure, which may be secondary to a space-occupying lesion, herniated disk, tumor, or osteophyte in the lumbar canal. Pain may be localized or referred to corresponding dermatome.

SPECIAL CONSIDERATIONS/COMMENTS:
The increased pressure may alter venous function and cause dizziness or unconsciousness. The examiner should be prepared to steady the subject.

LUMBAR SPINE

Stoop Test

TEST POSITIONING:
The subject is asked to walk briskly for a period of 1 minute.

ACTION:
The examiner assesses for the onset of pain in the buttock and lower limb areas. If present, the subject forward flexes the trunk.

POSITIVE FINDING:
Pain in the buttock and lower limb areas brought on by brisk walking that is soon relieved with forward flexing of the trunk is an indication that there is a relationship between the neurogenic intermittent claudication, posture, and walking.

SPECIAL CONSIDERATIONS/COMMENTS:
A positive test can be re-confirmed by positioning the patient back into trunk extension which may reproduce the painful symptoms.

Hoover Test

TEST POSITIONING:
The subject relaxes in a supine position on the table while the examiner places each heel of the subject's foot into the palm of the examiner's hands (Figure 64A).

ACTION:
The subject is asked to perform a unilateral straight leg raise (Figure 64B).

POSITIVE FINDING:
The inability to lift the leg may reflect a neuromuscular weakness. A positive finding is also noted when the examiner does not feel increased pressure in the palm that underlies the resting leg.

SPECIAL CONSIDERATIONS/COMMENTS:
Typically, when the raised leg is weak, pressure under the resting calcaneus will increase in an attempt to lift the weak leg. When this increase in pressure is not felt, it could indicate a lack of effort by the subject. This test should therefore be performed on both sides to test consistency of effort.

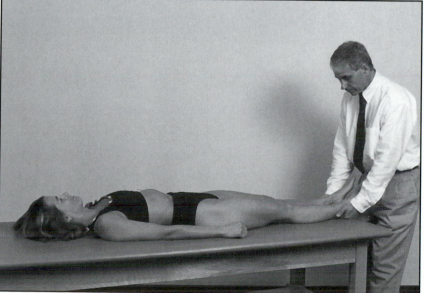

LUMBAR SPINE

FIGURE 64A

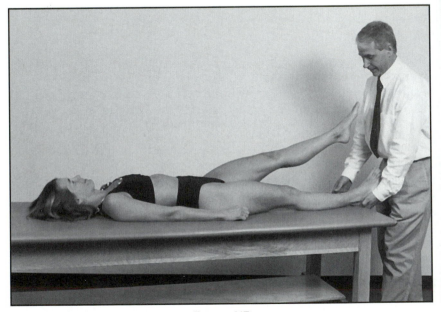

FIGURE 64B

Kernig/Brudzinski Test

TEST POSITIONING:
The subject is lying supine with the hands cupped behind the head. The examiner stands next to the subject.

ACTION:
The subject is instructed to flex the cervical spine by lifting the head. Each hip is unilaterally flexed to no more than 90 degrees by the subject. The subject then flexes the knee to no more than 90 degrees. The opposite leg remains on the examining table (Figure 65).

POSITIVE FINDING:
Increased pain, that may be localized or radiating into the lower extremity, with neck and hip flexion indicates a positive finding. The pain is relieved when the knee is flexed. The pain is indicative of meningeal irritation, nerve root impingement, or dural irritation that is exaggerated by elongating the spinal cord.

SPECIAL CONSIDERATIONS/COMMENTS:
Considerations are similar to the Straight Leg Raise Test except the neck is flexed and the hip is actively flexed. The neck flexion component of this test was developed by Kernig, whereas the hip flexion component was developed by Brudzinski.

LUMBAR SPINE

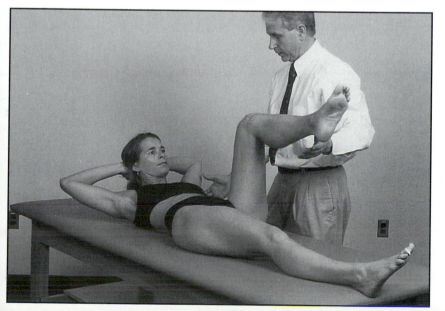

FIGURE 65

90-90 Straight Leg Raise Test

TEST POSITIONING:
The patient is lying supine, stabilizing both hips at 90 degrees of flexion with both hands. The knees are bent in a relaxed position. The examiner stands next to the patient (Figure 66A).

ACTION:
The patient is instructed to actively extend one knee at a time as much as possible (Figure 66B).

POSITIVE FINDING:
If the knee is flexed greater than 20 degrees, the hamstrings are considered tight.

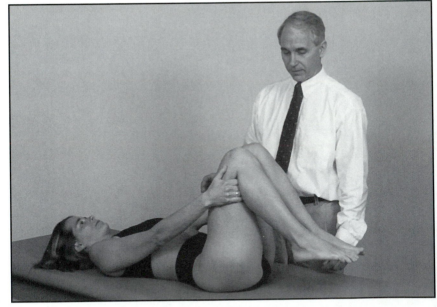

FIGURE 66A

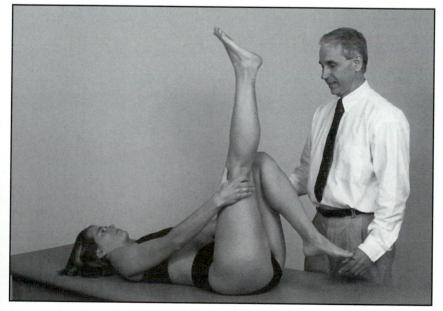

FIGURE 66B

Bowstring Test (Cram Test)

TEST POSITIONING:
The subject lies supine.

ACTION:
The examiner performs a passive straight leg raise on the involved side (Figure 67A). If the subject reports radiating pain with the straight leg raise, the examiner then flexes the subject's knee to approximately 20 degrees in an attempt to reduce painful symptoms. The examiner then applies pressure to the popliteal area in an attempt to reproduce the radicular pain (Figure 67B).

POSITIVE FINDING:
Painful radicular reproduction following popliteal compression indicates tension on the sciatic nerve.

SPECIAL CONSIDERATIONS/COMMENTS:
It is important for the examiner to maintain the same degree of the subject's hip flexion when flexion of the knee is performed.

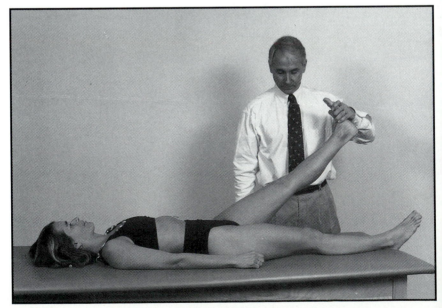

FIGURE 67A

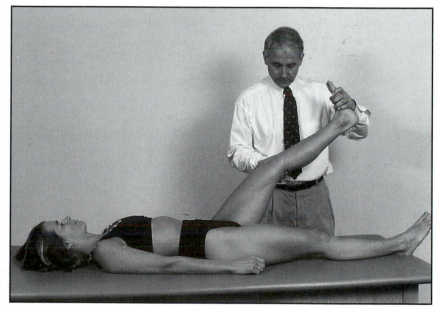

FIGURE 67B

Sitting Root Test

TEST POSITIONING:
The subject is seated with the hip flexed to 90 degrees and the cervical spine in flexion.

ACTION:
The subject actively extends the knee (Figure 68A).

POSITIVE FINDING:
The subject who arches backwards and/or complains of pain in the regions of the buttock, posterior thigh, and calf during knee extension demonstrates a positive finding for possible sciatic nerve pain.

SPECIAL CONSIDERATIONS/COMMENTS:
This test can be reproduced with the examiner passively extending the subject's knee. True sciatic pain should still cause the subject to react. However, if the examiner's actions distract the subject from being aware of the area being tested, the subject may respond differently. For example, if the examiner stabilized and visualized the foot during extension of the knee, the subject may be unaware that the examiner is really testing for sciatic tension (Figure 68B).

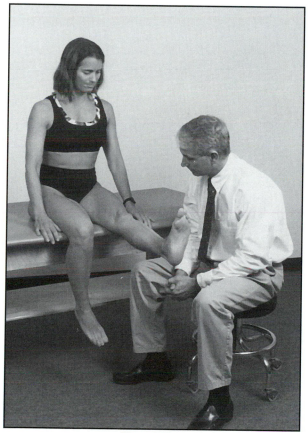

FIGURE 68A

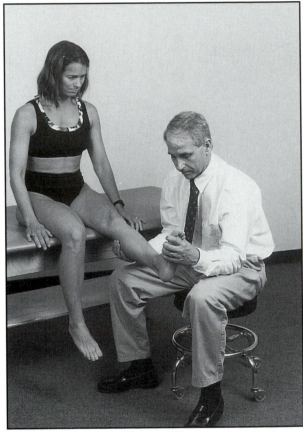

FIGURE 68B

Unilateral Straight Leg Raise (Lasegue) Test

TEST POSITIONING:
The subject is supine with both hips and knees extended. The examiner is standing with the distal hand around the subject's heel and the proximal hand on the subject's distal thigh (anteriorly) to maintain knee extension.

ACTION:
With the subject completely relaxed, slowly raise the test leg until pain or tightness is noted (Figure 69). Slowly lower the leg until the pain or tightness resolves, at which point dorsiflex the ankle and have the subject flex the neck.

POSITIVE FINDING:
Leg and/or low back pain occurring with dorsiflexion and/or neck flexion is indicative of dural involvement. A lack of pain reproduction with dorsiflexion and/or neck flexion is indicative of either hamstring tightness or possibly lumbar spine or sacroiliac joint involvement. Additionally, pain occurring at hip flexion angles >70 degrees is indicative of lumbar spine or sacroiliac joint involvement. If the latter is determined, proceed to the Bilateral Straight Leg Raise Test to differentiate between lumbar spine and sacroiliac joint involvement.

SPECIAL CONSIDERATIONS/COMMENTS:
The subject must be completely relaxed as contraction of the hip flexor muscles could increase the stress placed on the lumbar spine and sacroiliac joint, thus creating false positive findings. Additionally, during the Unilateral Straight Leg Raise Test, pain may be noted in the contralateral leg and/or lumbar spine. This finding should be referred to as a positive Crossed Straight Leg Raise Test.

LUMBAR SPINE

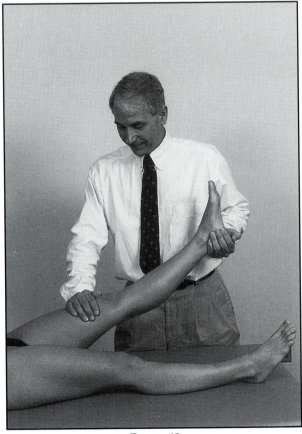

FIGURE 69

Bilateral Straight Leg Raise Test

TEST POSITIONING:
The subject is supine with both hips and knees extended. The examiner is standing with the distal hand or forearm around or under the subject's heels and the proximal hand on the subject's distal thighs (anteriorly) to maintain knee extension.

ACTION:
With the subject completely relaxed, slowly raise the legs until pain or tightness is noted (Figure 70).

POSITIVE FINDING:
Low back pain occurring at hip flexion angles <70 degrees is indicative of sacroiliac joint involvement. Low back pain occurring at hip flexion angles >70 degrees is indicative of lumbar spine involvement.

SPECIAL CONSIDERATIONS/COMMENTS:
The examiner must utilize proper body mechanics when performing this test in order to avoid injury secondary to lifting the weight of both legs.

LUMBAR SPINE

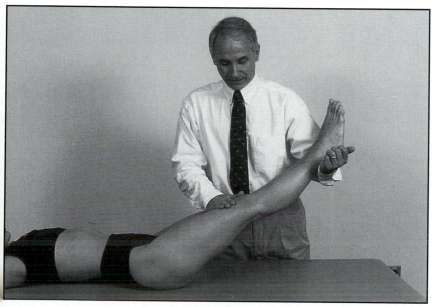

FIGURE 70

Thomas Test

TEST POSITIONING:
The subject is supine with both knees against the chest and the buttocks near the table edge. The examiner is standing with one hand on the subject's lumbar spine or iliac crest to monitor lumbar lordosis or pelvic tilt, respectively (Figure 71A).

ACTION:
The subject slowly lowers the test leg until the leg is fully relaxed or until either anterior pelvic tilting or an increase in lumbar lordosis occurs (Figure 71B).

POSITIVE FINDING:
A lack of hip extension with knee flexion >45 degrees is indicative of iliopsoas muscle tightness. Full hip extension with knee flexion <45 degrees is indicative of rectus femoris muscle tightness. A lack of hip extension with knee flexion <45 degrees is indicative of iliopsoas and rectus femoris muscle tightness. Hip external rotation during any of the previous scenarios is indicative of iliotibial band (particularly the tensor fascia latae) tightness.

SPECIAL CONSIDERATIONS/COMMENTS:
Increases in anterior pelvic tilt and lumbar lordosis must be eliminated in order to prevent false negative findings. To further confirm this assessment, the examiner can simply apply pressure on the lower leg in an effort to lower it back to the table. A return of lumbar lordosis will indicate a positive finding.

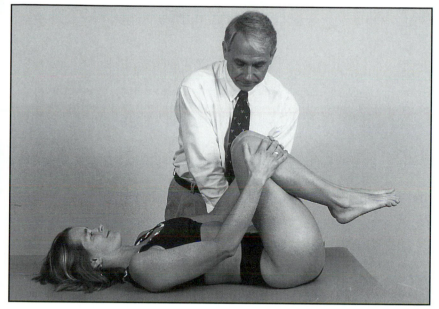

Figure 71A

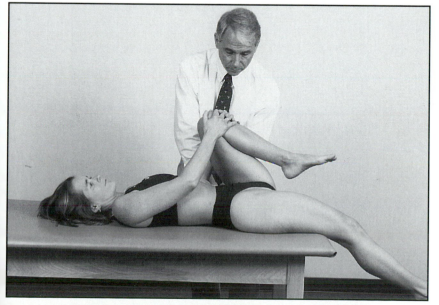

Figure 71B

Spring Test

TEST POSITIONING:
The subject is prone, and the examiner is standing with the thumb
(Figure 72A) or hypothenar eminence (specifically the pisiform) over
the spinous process of a lumbar vertebra (Figure 72B).

ACTION:
Apply a downward "springing" force through the spinous process of
each vertebra to assess anterior-posterior (A-P) motion. This action
should be repeated for each transverse process to assess rotary motion.

POSITIVE FINDING:
Increases or decreases in motion at one vertebra compared to another
are indicative of hypermobility or hypomobility, respectively.

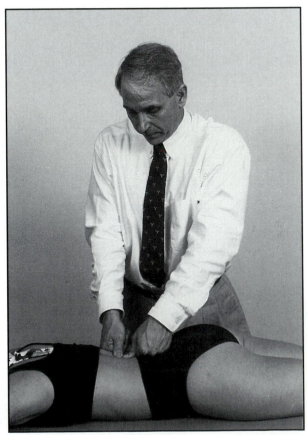

FIGURE 72A

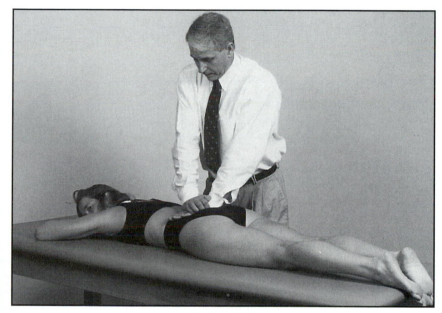

FIGURE 72B

Trendelenburg Test

TEST POSITIONING:
The subject stands on one lower extremity (Figures 73A and 73B).

ACTION:
The subject remains in this position for approximatly 10 seconds and then switches extremities.

POSITIVE FINDING:
A positive finding is seen when the pelvis on the unsupported side drops noticeably lower than the pelvis on the supported side. This indicates a weakness of the gluteus medius muscle on the supported side.

SPECIAL CONSIDERATIONS/COMMENTS:
With a negative test, the gluteus medius on the supported side will perform a reverse action since the supported femur is stabilized. This will allow for the unsupported pelvis to remain level with the supported pelvis. With a weak gluteus medius on the supported side, the unsupported pelvis drops as the muscles fatigues. This test may also indicate an unstable hip on the supported side.

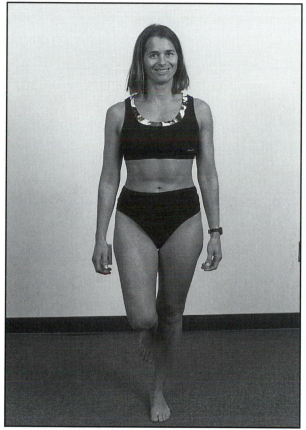

FIGURE 73A

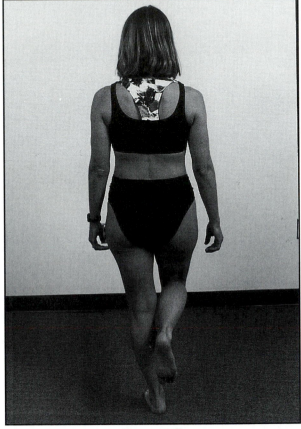

FIGURE 73B

SECTION IX

Sacral Spine

Sacroiliac (SI) Joint Fixation Test

TEST POSITIONING:
The subject is standing with the SI joint exposed.
1. The examiner stands behind the subject with the thumbs over the posterior superior iliac spines (Figure 74A).

ACTION:
1. The examiner should note whether the posterior superior iliac spines are level.

POSITIVE FINDING:
1. If the posterior superior iliac spines are not level, the SI joints are asymmetrical, indicating fixation on one side or the other.

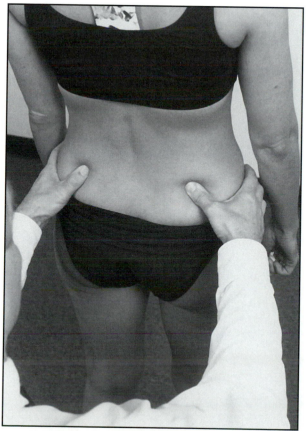

FIGURE 74A

TEST POSITIONING:
2. The examiner then places one thumb over the posterior superior iliac spine on the right or left side, and the other thumb over the S2 spinous process. Repeat on the other side (Figure 74B).

ACTION:
2. The subject is then instructed to actively flex each hip one at a time with the knee bent to 90 degrees. Compare to the other side (Figure 74C).

POSITIVE FINDING:
2. When the subject flexes each hip, the thumb over the posterior superior iliac spine should drop relative to the spinous process. If there is no change or the thumb moves superiorly, hypomobility is indicated.

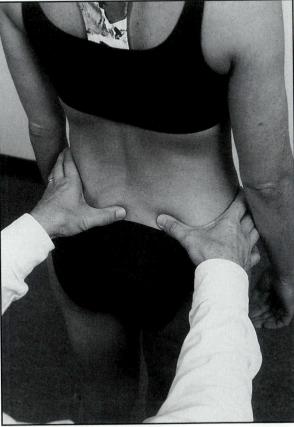

FIGURE 74B

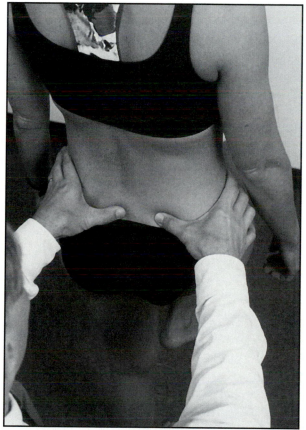

FIGURE 74C

TEST POSITIONING:

3. The examiner may then leave the one thumb over the sacral spinous process and move the other thumb to the ischial tuberosity. Repeat on the other side (Figure 74D).

ACTION:

3. The subject is instructed again to actively flex one hip at a time with the knee bent to 90 degrees. Compare to the other side (Figure 74E).

POSITIVE FINDING:

3. When the subject again flexes each hip, the thumb over the ischial tuberosity should move inferiorly. If the thumb moves superiorly, hypomobility is indicated.

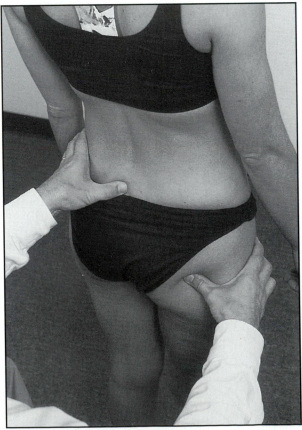

FIGURE 74D

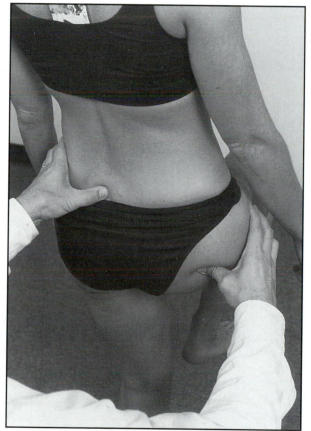

Figure 74E

Sacroiliac (SI) Joint Stress Test

TEST POSITIONING:
1. The subject is lying supine. The examiner stands next to the subject and, with the arms crossed, places the heel of both hands on the subject's anterior superior iliac spines (Figure 75A).

ACTION:
1. The examiner applies out and downward pressure with the heel of the hands.

POSITIVE FINDING:
1. Unilateral pain at the SI joint or in the gluteal or leg region indicates an anterior SI ligament sprain.

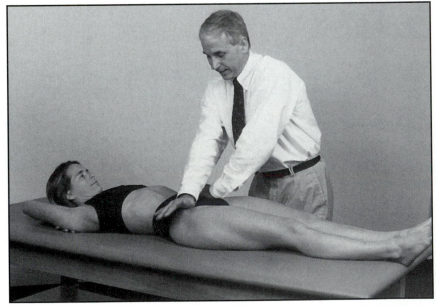

FIGURE 75A

Test Positioning:

2. The subject is side lying. The examiner stands next to the subject and places both hands, one on top of the other, directly over the subject's iliac crest. Repeat on the other side (Figure 75B).

Action:

2. The examiner applies downward pressure. Compare to the other side.

Positive Finding:

2. Increased pain or pressure is indicative of SI joint pathology, possibly involving the posterior SI ligaments.

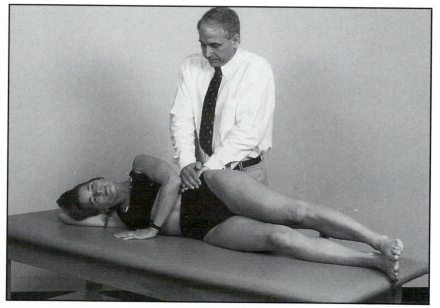

Figure 75B

TEST POSITIONING:
3. The subject is lying supine. The examiner places both hands on the lateral aspect of the subject's iliac crests (Figure 75C).

ACTION:
3. The examiner applies inward and downward pressure.

POSITIVE FINDING:
3. Increased pain or pressure is indicative of SI joint pathology, possibly involving the posterior SI ligaments.

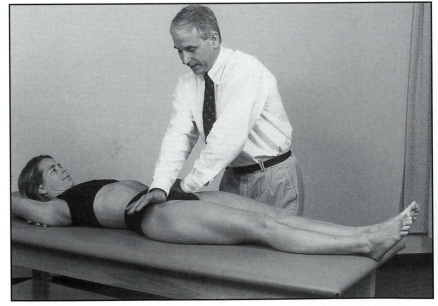

FIGURE 75C

Test Positioning:

4. The subject is lying prone. The examiner places both hands, one on top of the other, over the subjects' sacrum (Figure 75D).

Action:

4. The examiner applies downward pressure, creating a shear of the sacrum on the ilium.

Positive Finding:

4. Pain at the SI joint is indicative of SI joint pathology.

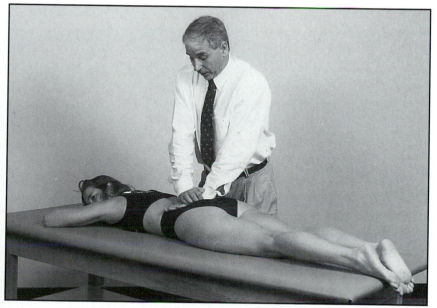

Figure 75D

Sacral Spine

Patrick or FABER Test

TEST POSITIONING:
The subject lies supine on the table.

ACTION:
The examiner passively flexes, abducts, and externally rotates the involved leg until the foot rests on the top of the knee of the non-involved lower extremity (Figure 76A). The examiner then slowly abducts the involved lower extremity toward the table (Figure 76B).

POSITIVE FINDING:
A positive finding is revealed when the involved lower extremity does not abduct below the level of the non-involved lower extremity. This may be indicative of iliopsoas, sacroiliac, or even hip joint abnormalities.

SPECIAL CONSIDERATIONS/COMMENTS:
"FABER" is reflective of the initial positioning of the subject (flexion = F, abduction = AB, external rotation = ER).

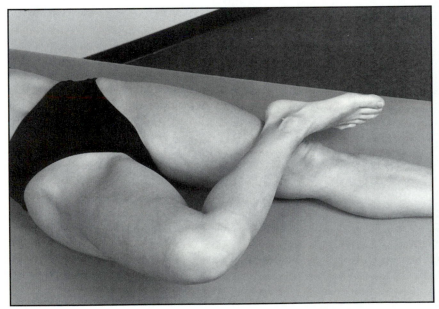

FIGURE 76A

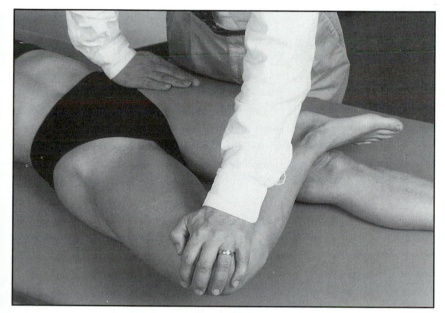

Figure 76B

Long-Sitting Test

TEST POSITIONING:
The subject is supine with both hips and knees extended, and the
 examiner is standing with the thumbs on the subject's medial malleoli
(Figure 77A).

ACTION:
The examiner passively flexes both knees and hips (Figure 77B) and
then fully extends and compares the position of the medial malleoli
relative to each other (Figure 77C). The subject then slowly assumes
the long-sitting position and malleolar position is re-assessed (Figure
77D).

POSITIVE FINDING:
A leg that appears longer in supine but shorter in long-sitting is indicative of an ipsilateral anteriorly rotated ilium. Conversely, a leg that
appears shorter in supine but longer in long-sitting is indicative of an
ipsilateral posteriorly rotated ilium.

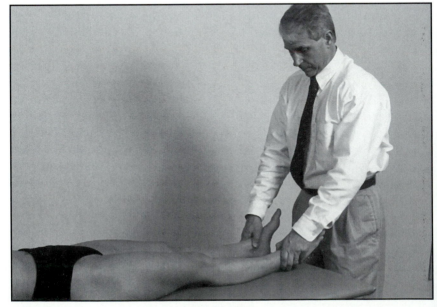

FIGURE 77A

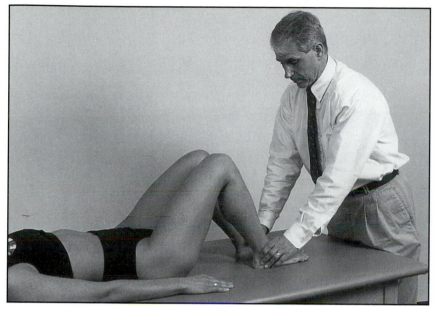

Figure 77B

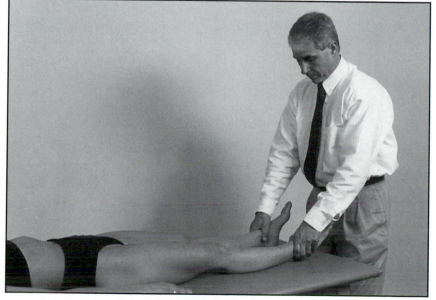

Figure 77C

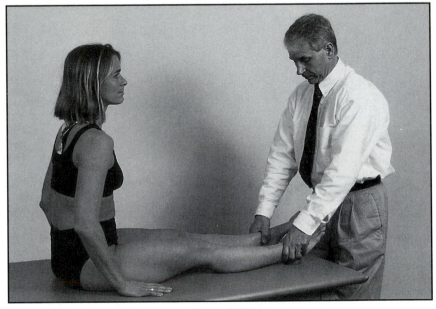

FIGURE 77D

SECTION X

Hip

Hip Scouring or Quadrant Test

TEST POSITIONING:
The subject is lying supine. The examiner stands on the involved side and passively flexes and adducts the subject's hip. The subject's knee is also placed in full flexion (Figure 78A).

ACTION:
The examiner applies downward pressure along the shaft of the femur while simultaneously adducting and externally rotating the hip (Figure 78B). The examiner then adducts and internally rotates the hip while maintaining downward pressure (Figure 78C). This movement is repeated two to three times while the examiner notes any unusual movement (ie, catching, grinding), or subject apprehension.

POSITIVE FINDING:
Pain or apprehension is indicative of hip joint pathology such as arthritis, osteochondral defects, avascular necrosis, or acetabular labrum defects.

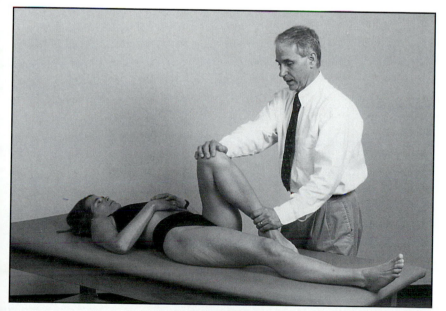

FIGURE 78A

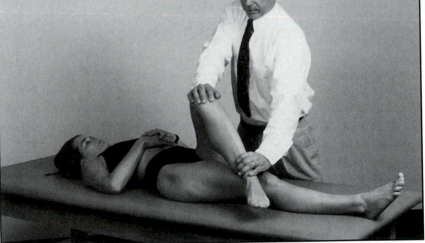

FIGURE 78B

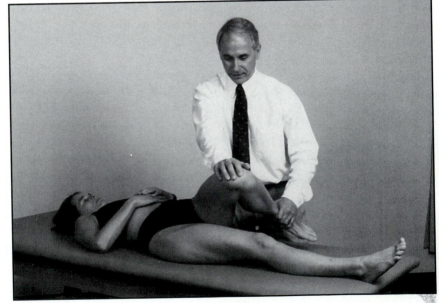

FIGURE 78C

Nelaton's Line

TEST POSITIONING:
The subject is lying supine with both legs extended. The examiner stands on the involved side and imagines a line from the subject's anterior superior iliac spine to the ischial tuberosity.

ACTION:
The position of the greater trochanter is palpated in relation to the line. This process is repeated on the other side for comparison (Figure 79).

POSITIVE FINDING:
If the greater trochanter is positioned above the imaginary line, coxa vara or a decreased angle of inclination is present. Coxa vara presents as a valgus posture at the knee and may lead to lower extremity malalignment and subsequent pathologies.

SPECIAL CONSIDERATIONS/COMMENTS:
If the greater trochanter is palpated well above the line, a dislocated hip may also be indicated.

Hip

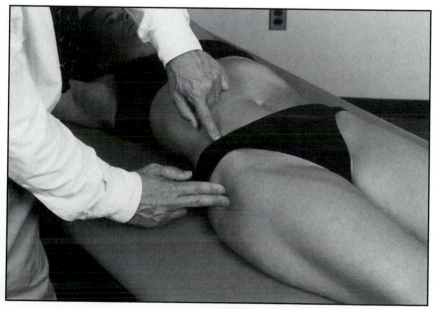

FIGURE 79

Craig's Test

TEST POSITIONING:
The subject is lying prone with the affected leg's knee flexed to 90 degrees. The examiner stands on the involved side and palpates the greater trochanter (Figure 80A).

ACTION:
The examiner then passively internally and externally rotates the femur until the greater trochanter is parallel with the examining table (Figure 80B). At this point, the subject is asked to hold the hip in this position while the examiner measures the angle between the long axis of the lower leg and the perpendicular axis to the table with a goniometer (Figure 80C).

POSITIVE FINDING:
If the measured angle is greater than 15 degrees, femoral anteversion is indicated. If the measured angle is less than 8 degrees, femoral retroversion is indicated. Increased femoral anteversion leads to toeing-in and squinting patellae. Femoral retroversion leads to a toeing-out position. Both of these may lead to lower extremity malalignment and subsequent pathologies.

SPECIAL CONSIDERATIONS/COMMENTS:
A second examiner may be useful to hold the subject's hip and leg in the designated position, while the first examiner measures the angle. This test is also known as the Ryder method for measuring femoral anteversion and retroversion.

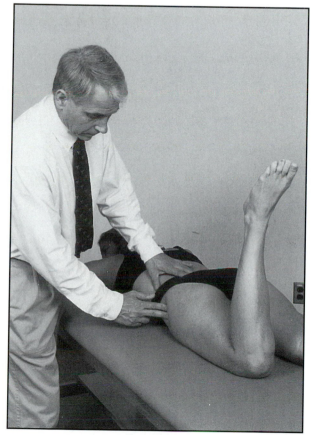

FIGURE 80A

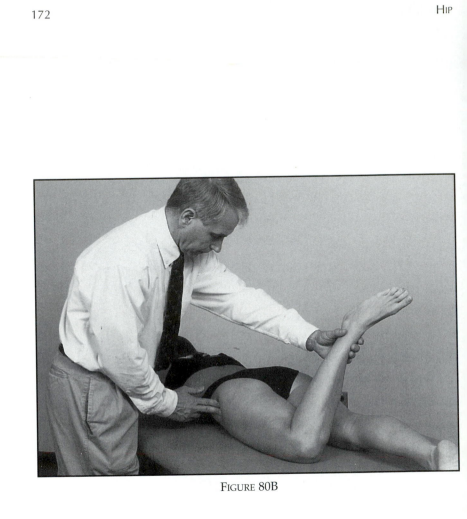

FIGURE 80B

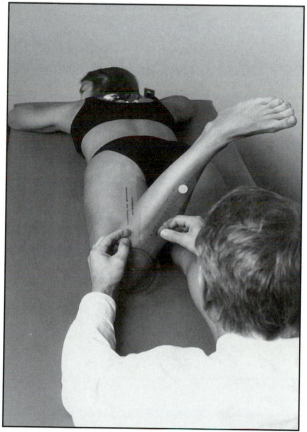

FIGURE 80C

90-90 Straight Leg Raise Test

TEST POSITIONING:
The subject is lying supine, stabilizing both hips at 90 degrees of flexion with both hands. The knees are bent in a relaxed position. The examiner stands next to the subject (Figure 81A).

ACTION:
The subject is instructed to actively extend one knee at a time as much as possible (Figure 81B).

POSITIVE FINDING:
If the knee is flexed greater than 20 degrees, the hamstrings are considered tight.

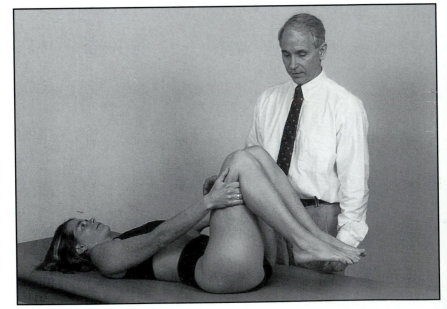

FIGURE 81A

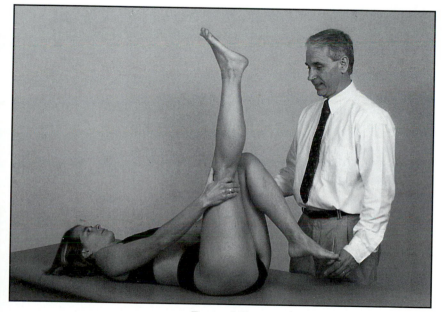

FIGURE 81B

Patrick or FABER Test

TEST POSITIONING:
The subject lies supine on the table.

ACTION:
The examiner passively flexes, abducts, and externally rotates the involved leg until the foot rests on the top of the knee of the non-involved lower extremity (Figure 82A). The examiner then slowly abducts the involved lower extremity toward the table (Figure 82B).

POSITIVE FINDING:
A positive finding is revealed when the involved lower extremity does not abduct below the level of the non-involved lower extremity. This may be indicative of iliopsoas, sacro-iliac, or even hip joint abnormalities.

SPECIAL CONSIDERATIONS/COMMENTS:
"FABER" is reflective of the initial positioning of the subject (flexion = F, abduction = AB, external rotation = ER).

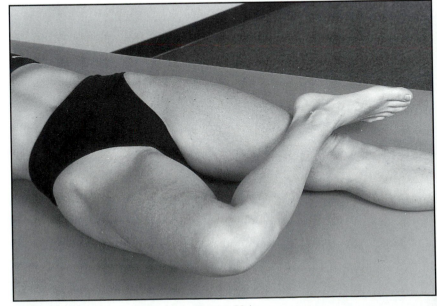

FIGURE 82A

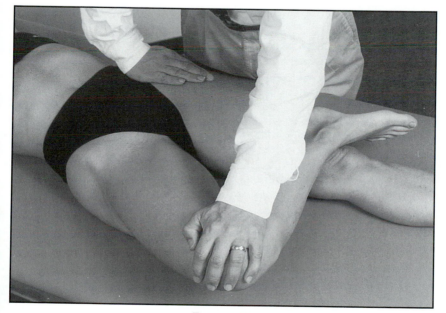

FIGURE 82B

Trendelenburg Test

TEST POSITIONING:
The subjects stands on one lower extremity (Figures 83A and 83B).

ACTION:
The subject remains in this position for approximately 10 seconds and then switches extremities.

POSITIVE FINDING:
A positive finding is seen when the pelvis on the unsupported side drops noticeably lower than the pelvis on the supported side. This indicates a weakness of the gluteus medius muscle on the supported side.

SPECIAL CONSIDERATIONS/COMMENTS:
With a negative test, the gluteus medius on the supported side will perform a reverse action since the supported femur is stabilized. This will allow for the unsupported pelvis to remain level with the supported pelvis. With a weak gluteus medius on the supported side, the unsupported pelvis drops as the muscle fatigues. This test may also indicate an unstable hip on the supported side.

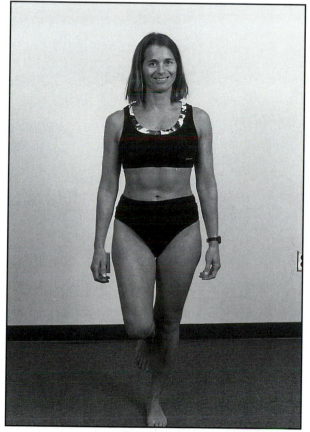

FIGURE 83A

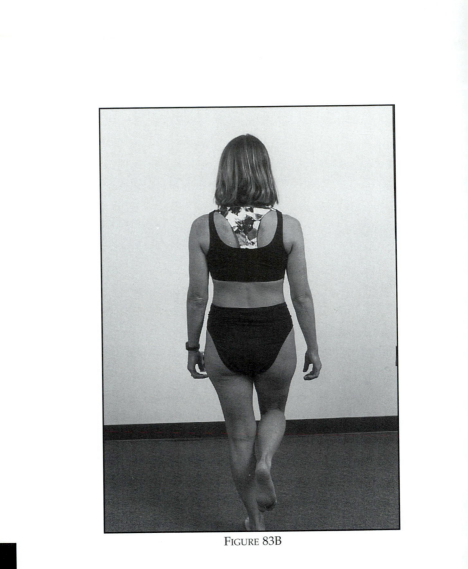

FIGURE 83B

Ober Test

TEST POSITIONING:
The subject is side lying with the hips and knees extended such that the test leg is superior to the non-test leg. The examiner is standing with the proximal hand stabilizing the pelvis and the distal hand supporting the lower leg (Figure 84A).

ACTION:
With the pelvis stabilized to prevent rolling, abduct and extend the test hip in order to position the iliotibial band (ITB) behind the greater trochanter (Figure 84B). Then allow the leg to slowly lower (adduct).

POSITIVE FINDING:
The inability of the leg to adduct and touch the table is indicative of ITB (particularly the tensor fasciae latae) tightness. The leg will react like a "springboard" since the leg remains abducted in mid-air.

SPECIAL CONSIDERATIONS/COMMENTS:
It is important to apply a downward force on the ilium near the crest while allowing the leg to adduct. This will prevent lateral tilting (ie, inferior movement) of the pelvis on the side of the test leg, which could give a false negative. Additionally, it is important to ensure complete relaxation of the hip abductor muscles. It may be helpful to have the subject actively adduct the test leg into the support hand and then relax in order to inhibit hip abductor muscle guarding.

Hip

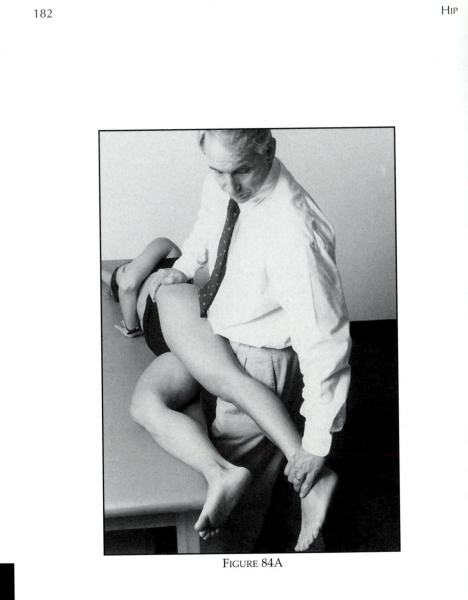

FIGURE 84A

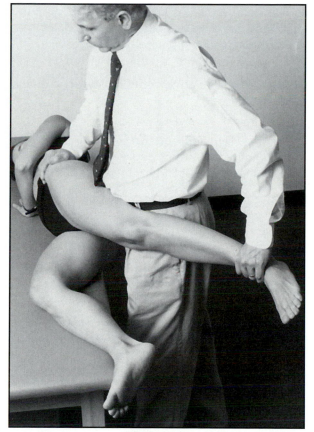

FIGURE 84B

Piriformis Test

TEST POSITIONING:
The subject is side lying on the non-test side with the test leg in 60 degrees of hip flexion and relaxed knee flexion. The examiner is standing with the proximal hand on the subject's pelvis (laterally) and the distal hand on the subject's knee (laterally) (Figure 85).

ACTION:
With the subject's pelvis stabilized, apply an adduction (downward) force on the subject's knee.

POSITIVE FINDING:
Tightness or pain in the hip and buttock areas is indicative of piriformis tightness. Pain in the buttock and posterior thigh is indicative of sciatic nerve impingement secondary to piriformis tightness.

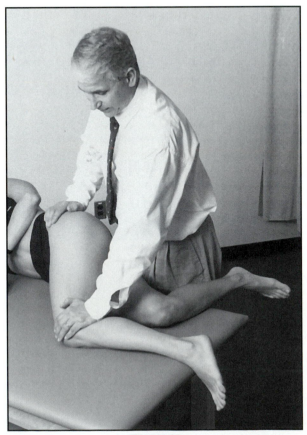

FIGURE 85

Thomas Test

TEST POSITIONING:
The subject is supine with both knees against the chest and the buttocks near the table edge. The examiner is standing with one hand on the subject's lumbar spine or iliac crest to monitor lumbar lordosis or pelvic tilt, respectively (Figure 86A).

ACTION:
The subject slowly lowers the test leg until the leg is fully relaxed or until either anterior pelvic tilting or an increase in lumbar lordosis occurs (Figure 86B).

POSITIVE FINDING:
A lack of hip extension with knee flexion >45 degrees is indicative of iliopsoas muscle tightness. Full hip extension with knee flexion <45 degrees is indicative of rectus femoris muscle tightness. A lack of hip extension with knee flexion <45 degrees is indicative of iliopsoas and rectus femoris muscle tightness. Hip external rotation during any of the previous scenarios is indicative of ITB (particularly the tensor fascia latae) tightness.

SPECIAL CONSIDERATIONS/COMMENTS:
Increases in anterior pelvic tilt and lumbar lordosis must be eliminated in order to prevent false negative findings. To further confirm this assessment, the examiner can simply apply pressure on the lower leg in an effort to lower it back to the table. A return of lumbar lordosis will indicate a positive finding.

Hip

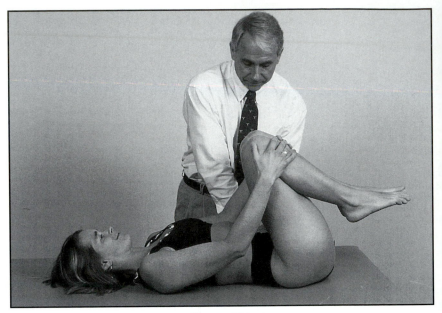

FIGURE 86A

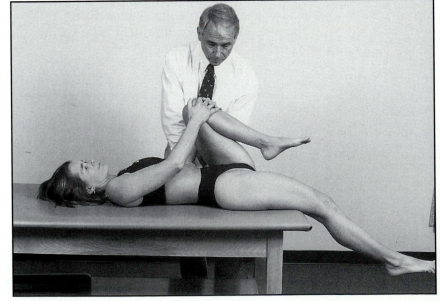

FIGURE 86B

True Leg Length Discrepancy Test

TEST POSITIONING:
The subject is supine with hips and knees extended and parallel with each other. Each leg should be perpendicular to a straight line between both anterior superior iliac spines (ASIS).

ACTION:
With a tape measure, measure from the most distal point of the ASIS to the most distal point of the medial malleolus (Figure 87).

POSITIVE FINDINGS:
A difference of >1 cm is indicative of discrepancies in either the length of the femur or tibia, or in the angle of femoral neck inclination (ie, coxa vara or valga).

SPECIAL CONSIDERATIONS/COMMENTS:
Significant discrepancies should be verified via radiography, as this is the most accurate method of assessing true leg length discrepancies.

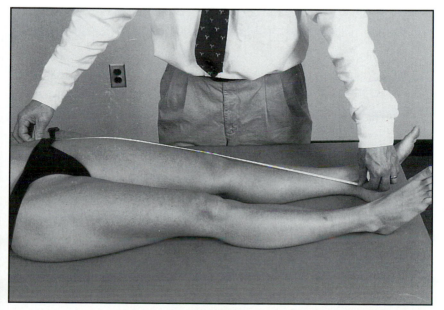

FIGURE 87

Ely's Test

TEST POSITIONING:
The subject is lying prone. The examiner stands on one side of the table next to the subject's leg.

ACTION:
The examiner passively flexes the subject's knee and notes the reaction at the hip joint. This test is repeated on the other side for comparison (Figure 88A).

POSITIVE FINDING:
When the knee is flexed, if the hip also flexes, a tight rectus femoris is indicated (Figure 88B).

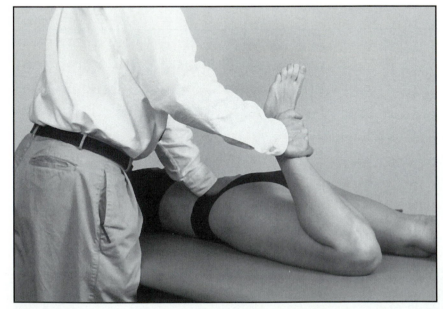

FIGURE 88A

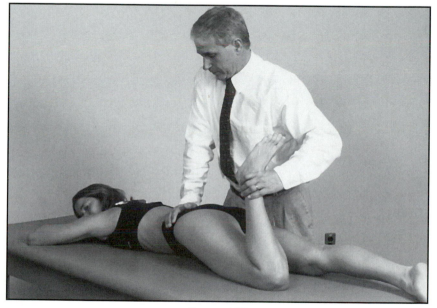

FIGURE 88B

Patella Tendon/
Patella Ligament Length Test

TEST POSITIONING:
The subject is supine on a table.

ACTION:
The examiner measures the distance between the superior pole of the patella to the inferior pole of the patella. The examiner next measures the distance between the inferior pole of the patella and the tibial tubercle (Figures 89A and 89B).

POSITIVE FINDING:
A ratio is taken between the first and the second measurement. A ratio of greater than 1 indicates patella baja, while a ratio of less than 1 indicates patella alta.

SPECIAL CONSIDERATIONS/COMMENTS:
Patella baja and patella alta may predispose one to various knee pathologies.

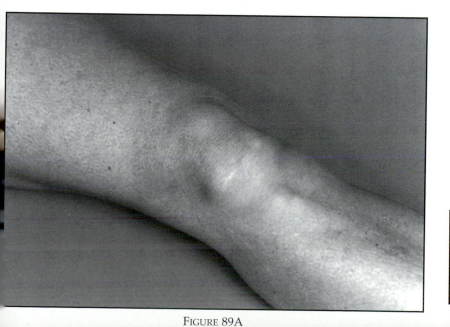

FIGURE 89A

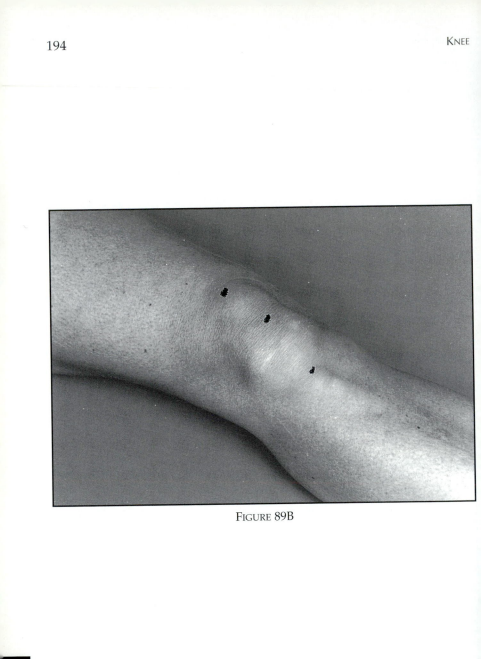

FIGURE 89B

PATELLAR APPREHENSION TEST

Patellar Apprehension Test

TEST POSITIONING:
The subject is lying supine with the knees extended. The examiner stands opposite to the involved side and places both thumbs on the medial border of the patella being tested (Figure 90A).

ACTION:
The subject must remain relaxed, while the examiner gently pushes the patella laterally.

POSITIVE FINDING:
If the subject is apprehensive to this movement, or the subject contracts the quadriceps muscle to protect against subluxation, the test is indicative of patellar subluxation or dislocation possibly due to laxity of the medial retinaculum.

SPECIAL CONSIDERATIONS/COMMENTS:
The action may be repeated with the knee flexed to 30 degrees (Figure 90B). The examiner must avoid excessive lateral patellar glide in order to prevent patellar dislocation.

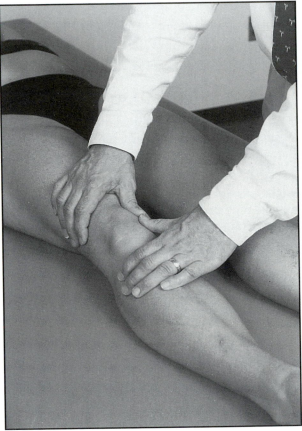

FIGURE 90A

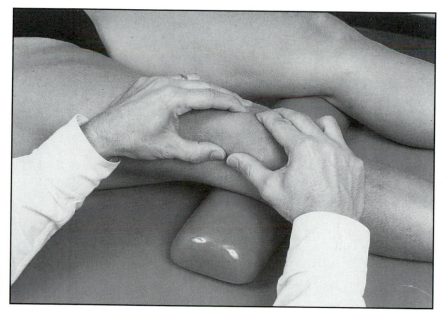

Figure 90B

Ballotable Patella or Patella Tap Test

TEST POSITIONING:
The subject is supine, and the examiner is standing with the proximal hand over the suprapatellar pouch and the distal hand (thumb or first two fingers) over the patella (Figure 91).

ACTION:
Compress the suprapatellar pouch with the proximal hand and then compress the patella into the femur.

POSITIVE FINDING:
Downward movement of the patella followed by a rebound will give the appearance of a floating or ballotable patella and is indicative of moderate to severe joint effusion.

SPECIAL CONSIDERATIONS/COMMENTS:
If a ballotable patella is determined, the examiner should take girth measurements at the supra-, mid-, and infrapatellar regions and compare bilaterally to more accurately assess the severity/degree of effusion. Additionally, the examiner must not mistake prepatellar bursitis as a joint effusion. The former will present as a "raw egg" over the patella but no downward patellar movement will be present. Occasionally, concomitant joint effusion and pre-patellar bursitis will present and the examiner will therefore be challenged to make the proper assessment.

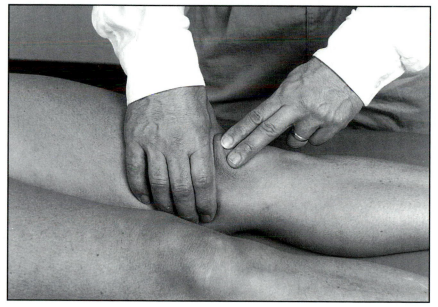

FIGURE 91

Quadriceps or Q-Angle Test

TEST POSITIONING:
The subject is supine with the hips and knees extended.

ACTION:
Identify the ASIS, midpoint of the patella, and the tibial tubercle. Strike a line from the ASIS to the midpoint of the patella, and from the tibial tubercle to the midpoint of the patella. Place a goniometer on the knee such that the axis is over the midpoint of the patella, the proximal arm is over the line to the ASIS, and the distal arm is over the line to the tibial tubercle. The resultant angle is the Q-Angle (Figure 92).

POSITIVE FINDING:
Q-angle norms with the knee in extension are 13 degrees for males and 18 degrees for females. Angles either greater than or less than these norms may be indicative of, but alone are not always accurate in predicting, patellofemoral pathology.

SPECIAL CONSIDERATIONS/COMMENTS:
Dynamic Q-angle measurements may be more indicative of patellofemoral function and underlying lower extremity pathomechanics than static Q-angle measurements.

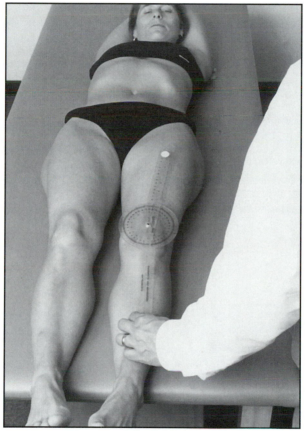

FIGURE 92

Medial-Lateral Grind Test

TEST POSITIONING:
The subject is lying supine. The examiner stands next to the involved side and holds the subject's foot. The examiner's other hand is placed over the joint line of the knee (Figure 93A).

ACTION:
The examiner passively flexes the subject's hip and knee maximally (Figure 93B), and then applies a circular motion with the tibia, rotating the tibia clockwise and counter-clockwise (Figure 93C).

POSITIVE FINDING:
Pain, grinding, or clicking is indicative of a meniscus tear.

SPECIAL CONSIDERATIONS:
Varus and valgus stress may be simultaneously applied by the hand over the joint line as the knee is passively extended (Anderson Medial-Lateral Grind).

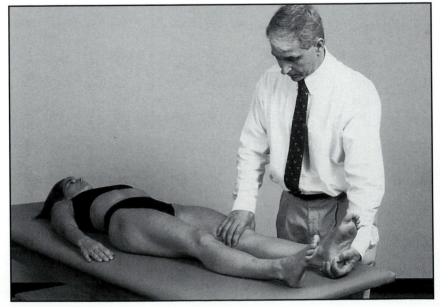

FIGURE 93A

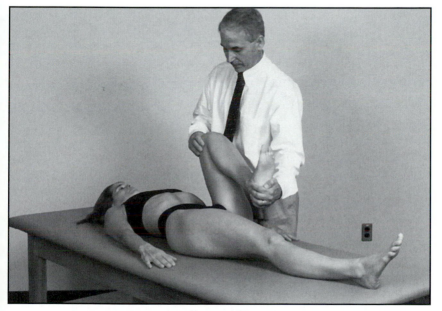

FIGURE 93B

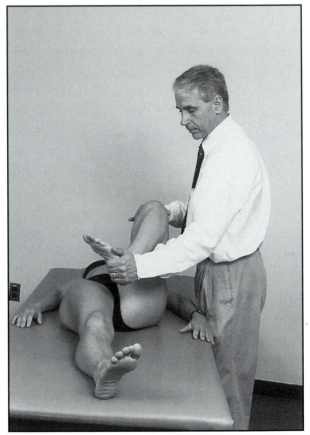

FIGURE 93C

Bounce Home Test

TEST POSITIONING:
The subject is lying supine. The examiner stands next to the involved side and cups the subject's foot in one hand. The examiner's other hand may be placed over the joint line of the knee (Figure 94A).

ACTION:
The examiner passively flexes the subject's knee (Figure 94B), then allows the knee to fall passively into extension (Figure 94C).

POSITIVE FINDING:
A rubbery end-feel or springy block is indicative of a meniscal tear.

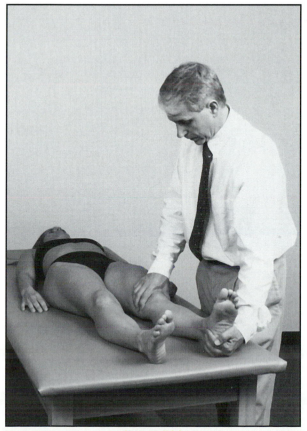

FIGURE 94A

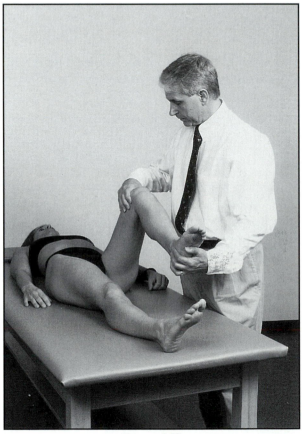

FIGURE 94B

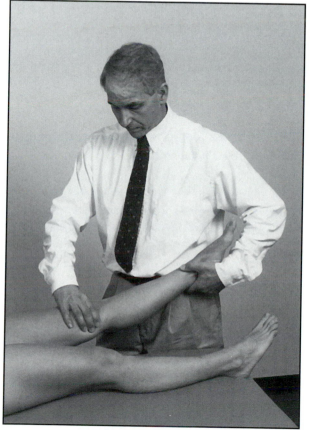

FIGURE 94C

Patellar Grind Test

TEST POSITIONING:
The subject is lying supine with the knees extended. The examiner stands next to the involved side and places the web space of the thumb on the superior border of the patella (Figure 95A).

ACTION:
The subject is asked to contract the quadriceps muscle, while the examiner applies downward and inferior pressure on the patella (Figure 95B).

POSITIVE FINDING:
Pain with movement of the patella or an inability to complete the test is indicative of chondromalacia patella.

SPECIAL CONSIDERATIONS/COMMENTS:
This test may be painful even for healthy subjects; therefore, it is important to bilaterally compare. This test may be repeated with the subject's knee in 30 degrees and 60 degrees of flexion to assess varying surfaces of the patella.

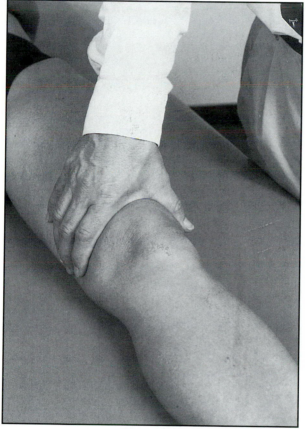

FIGURE 95A

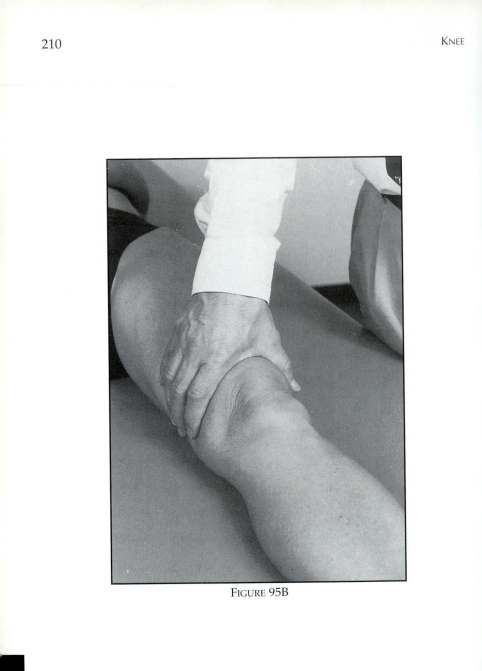

FIGURE 95B

Renne Test

TEST POSITIONING:
The subject is standing. The examiner stands in front of the subject and places the thumb over the lateral epicondyle of the involved knee (Figure 96A).

ACTION:
The subject is instructed to support the body weight on the involved foot and actively flex the knee as if performing a squat. The examiner maintains pressure with the thumb over the lateral epicondyle (Figure 96B).

POSITIVE FINDING:
If pain is present under the examiner's thumb when the subject's knee is positioned in 30 degrees of flexion, ITB friction syndrome is indicated.

SPECIAL CONSIDERATIONS/COMMENTS:
At 30 degrees of knee flexion, the ITB lies directly over the lateral epicondyle.

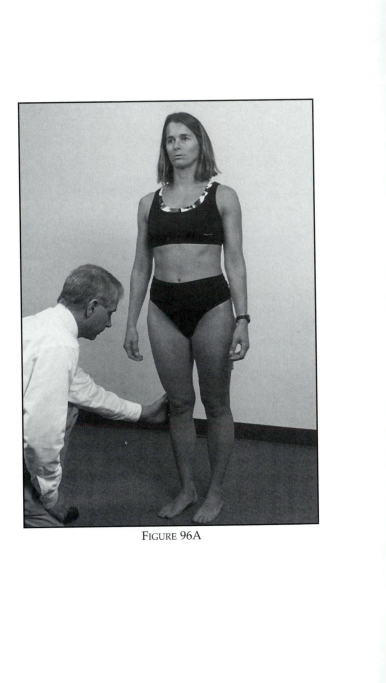

FIGURE 96A

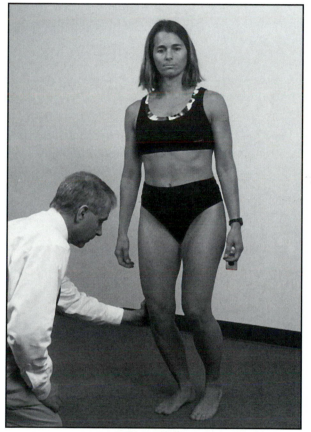

FIGURE 96B

Noble Test

TEST POSITIONING:
The subject is lying supine with the knee in flexion up to 90 degrees.
The examiner stands on the involved side and places the thumb over
the lateral epicondyle of the involved knee. The other hand is placed
around the subject's ankle.

ACTION:
The examiner passively extends and flexes the subject's knee while
maintaining pressure over the lateral epicondyle (Figures 97A and 97B).

POSITIVE FINDING:
If pain is present under the examiner's thumb when the subject's knee is
positioned in 30 degrees of flexion, ITB friction syndrome is indicated.

SPECIAL CONSIDERATIONS/COMMENTS:
At 30 degrees of knee flexion the ITB lies directly over the lateral epicondyle.

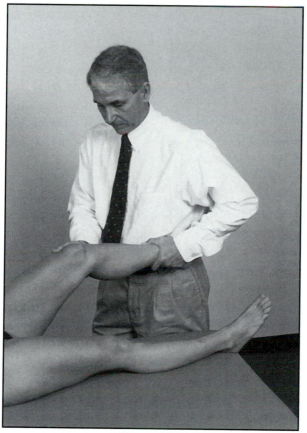

Figure 97A

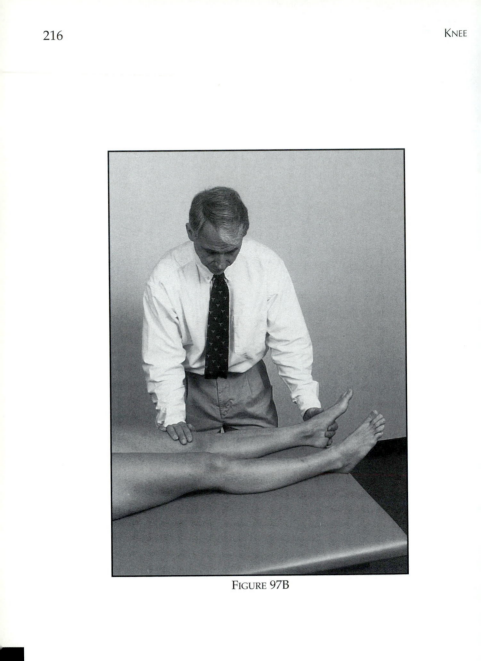

FIGURE 97B

Hughston's Plica Test

TEST POSITIONING:
The subject is lying supine with the involved knee extended and relaxed. The examiner stands on the involved side and places the heel of one hand over the lateral border of the patella, with the fingers of that hand positioned over the medial femoral condyle. The examiner's other hand is placed around the subject's ankle and foot (Figure 98A).

ACTION:
The examiner passively flexes and extends the subject's knee, while internally rotating the tibia and simultaneously pushing the patella medially (Figure 98B).

POSITIVE FINDING:
Pain and/or popping over the medial aspect of the knee is indicative of an abnormal plica.

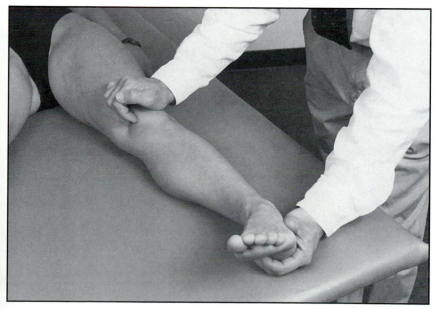

FIGURE 98A

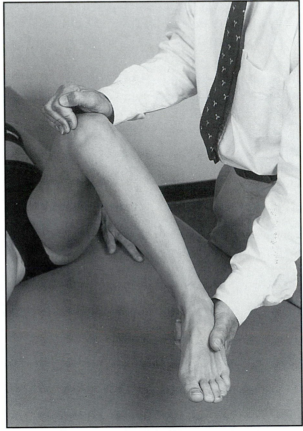

FIGURE 98B

Godfrey 90/90

TEST POSITIONING:
The subjects lies supine on a table with both the hip and knee of the involved side flexed to 90 degrees.

ACTION:
The examiner passively stabilizes the positioning of the subject's hip and knee while assessing the location of the tibia along the longitudinal axis (Figure 99).

POSITIVE FINDING:
The recognition of one tibia resting more inferior than the contralateral side may indicate a posterior sag or instability. This may be related to the posterior cruciate ligament.

SPECIAL CONSIDERATIONS/COMMENTS:
This test must be performed bilaterally. Applying a superior force to the tibia from the posterior aspect of the tibia may reduce the alignment to a normal resting position if it is actually found to be sagging.

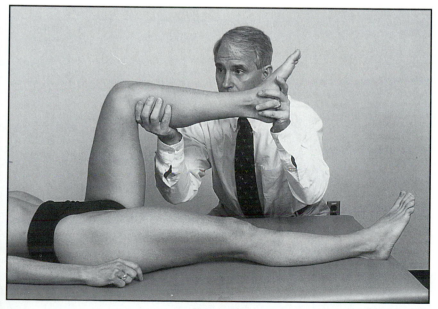

FIGURE 99

Posterior Sag Test
(Gravity Drawer Test)

TEST POSITIONING:
The subject lies on a a table with the involved knee flexed to 90 degrees
and the ipsilateral hip placed in 45 degrees of flexion (Figure 100).

ACTION:
The examiner observes the position of the tibia relative to the femur in
the sagittal plane. The examiner then instructs the subject to actively
contract the quadriceps muscle group in an attempt to extend the knee
while retaining hip flexion. The ipsilateral foot should remain fixated
to the table during the attempted knee extension.

POSITIVE FINDING:
Posterior displacement of the tibia upon the femur while the subject's
quadriceps remain silent indicates a posterior instability. This may be
reflective of injury to any of the following structures: posterior cruciate
ligament, arcuate ligament complex, and posterior oblique ligament.

SPECIAL CONSIDERATIONS/COMMENTS:
It is imperative for the examiner to identify a neutral tibio-femoral joint
position as this test can be misinterpreted for an anterior instability
when one observes an anterior translation of the tibia on the femur.

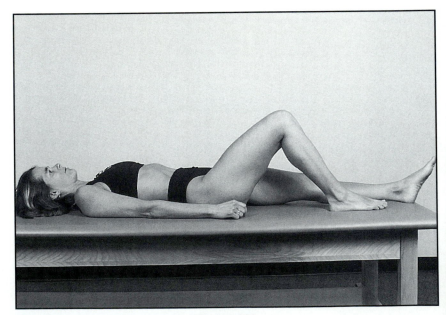

FIGURE 100

Reverse Pivot Shift (Jakob Test)

Test Positioning:
The subject is supine with the test knee in 40 to 50 degrees of flexion. The examiner is standing with the proximal hand on the subject's posterolateral leg just distal to the patella, with the thumb on or anterior to the fibular head and the distal hand grasping the subject's midfoot and heel (Figure 101A).
Alternate Test Positioning: Place the subject's foot between the examiner's distal arm and body with the same hand on the tibia and the proximal hand on the posterolateral leg just distal to the knee with the thumb on or anterior to the fibular head.

Action:
The examiner externally rotates the tibia with one hand and applies a valgus force with the other hand while slowly extending the knee. The same procedure applies for the alternate test position except apply a slight axial load as the knee is extended (Figure 101B).

Positive Finding:
This is first seen when the examiner flexes the subject's knee if the lateral tibial plateau subluxes posteriorly. Furthermore, this subluxation is reduced once the knee extends and approaches a position of approximately 20 degrees of flexion. At this point, the lateral tibial plateau will return to a neutral position. A palpable "clunk" or shift as it approaches extension (~20 to 30 degrees of flexion) is indicative of posterolateral rotary instability secondary to damage of primarily the PCL, LCL, posterolateral capsule, and arcuate complex.

Special Considerations/Comments:
This test is very sensitive to the subject who possesses an instability. It should be done only with the subject relaxed, as a contraction of the surrounding musculature of the knee may prevent a subtle subluxation, thus indicating a negative test.

KNEE

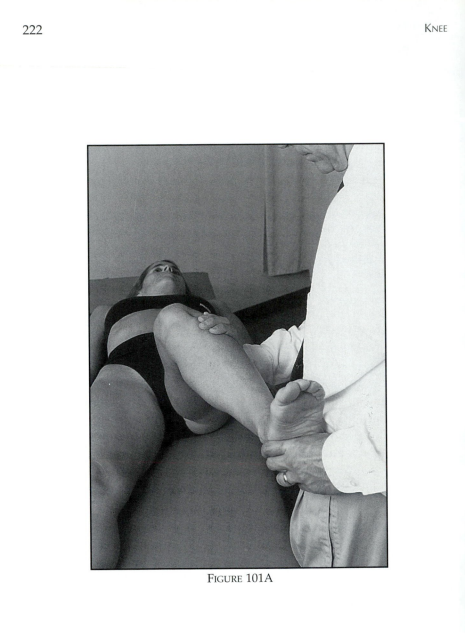

FIGURE 101A

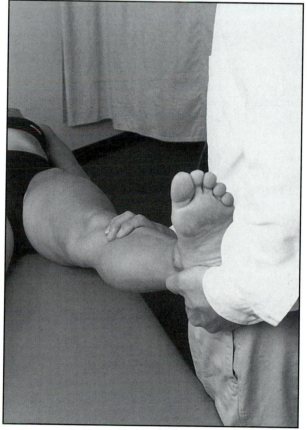

FIGURE 101B

Anterior Lachman Test

TEST POSITIONING:
The subject is supine with the test knee flexed to 20 to 30 degrees. The examiner is standing with the proximal hand on the subject's distal thigh (laterally) just proximal to patella, and the distal hand on the subject's proximal tibia (medially) just distal to tibial tubercle (Figure102A).
Alternate Test Positioning: The examiner places his or her flexed knee under the patient's test knee, proximal hand over the distal thigh (anteriorly) and distal hand on the subject's proximal tibia (medially), just distal to the tibial tubercle (Figure 102B).

ACTION:
From a "neutral" (anterior-posterior) position, apply an anterior force to the tibia with the distal hand while stabilizing the femur with the proximal hand. The same procedure applies for the alternate test positioning.

POSITIVE FINDING:
Excessive anterior translation of the tibia as compared to the uninvolved knee with a diminished or absent endpoint is indicative of a partial or complete tear of the anterior cruciate ligament.

SPECIAL CONSIDERATIONS/COMMENTS:
Increased anterior tibial translation is not in and of itself indicative of ACL pathology. For example, a torn PCL will allow the proximal tibia to translate posteriorly, thus producing increased anterior translation during the Anterior Lachman Test. Therefore, the presence and quality of the endpoint must be determined before ACL integrity may be accurately assessed.

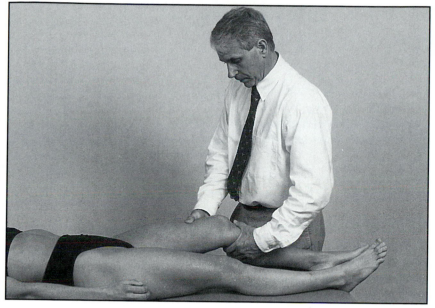

FIGURE 102A

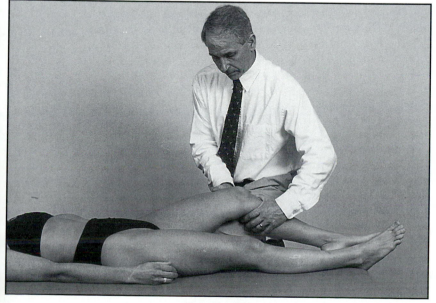

FIGURE 102B

Anterior Drawer Test

TEST POSITIONING:
The subject is supine with the test hip flexed to 45 degrees, knee flexed
to 90 degrees, and the foot in a neutral position. The examiner is sitting
on the subject's foot, with both hands behind the subject's proximal
tibia and thumbs on the tibial plateau (Figure 103).

ACTION:
Apply an anterior force to the proximal tibia. The hamstrings tendons
should be palpated frequently with index fingers to ensure relaxation.

POSITIVE FINDING:
Increased anterior tibial displacement as compared to the uninvolved
side is indicative of a partial or complete tear of the ACL.

SPECIAL CONSIDERATIONS/COMMENTS:
See "Special Considerations/Comments" for the Anterior Lachman
Test. Qualitative assessment of the endpoint during the Anterior
Drawer Test is less accurate than during the Anterior Lachman Test.
Also, a greater potential for false negative exists with this test versus
the Anterior Lachman Test, secondary to the increased potential for
hamstrings "guarding."

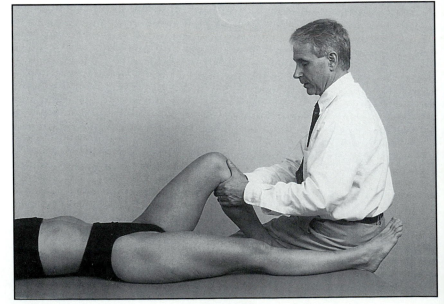

FIGURE 103

Slocum Test with Internal Tibial Rotation

TEST POSITIONING:
The subject is supine with the test hip flexed to 45 degrees, knee flexed to 90 degrees, and tibia internally rotated 15 to 20 degrees. The examiner is sitting on the subject's foot, with both hands behind the subject's proximal tibia and thumbs on the tibial plateau (Figure 104).

ACTION:
Apply an anterior force to the proximal tibia. The hamstrings tendons should be palpated frequently with index fingers to ensure relaxation.

POSITIVE FINDING:
Increased anterior tibial displacement, particularly of the lateral tibial condyle, as compared to the uninvolved side is indicative of anterolateral rotary instability, secondary to a partial or complete tear of primarily the ACL and posterolateral capsule.

SPECIAL CONSIDERATIONS/COMMENTS:
The examiner must avoid maximally rotating the tibia as this will tighten most of the surrounding structures, creating a high potential for false "negative" findings.

KNEE

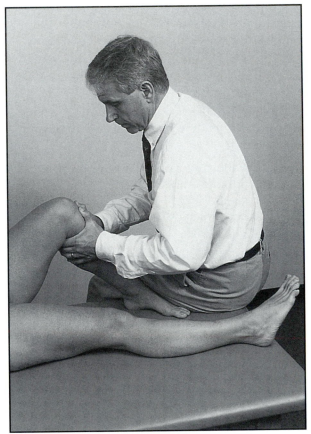

FIGURE 104

Slocum Test with External Tibial Rotation

TEST POSITIONING:

The subject is supine with the test hip flexed to 45 degrees, knee flexed to 90 degrees, and tibia externally rotated 15 to 20 degrees. The examiner is sitting on the subject's foot with both hands behind the subject's proximal tibia and thumbs on the tibial plateau (Figure 105).

ACTION:

Apply an anterior force to the proximal tibia. The hamstrings tendons should be palpated frequently with the index fingers to ensure relaxation.

POSITIVE FINDING:

Increased anterior tibial displacement, particularly of the medial tibial condyle, as compared to the uninvolved side is indicative of anteromedial rotary instability, secondary to damage to primarily the MCL, ACL, and posteromedial capsule.

SPECIAL CONSIDERATIONS/COMMENTS:

The examiner must avoid maximally rotating the tibia as this will tighten most of the surrounding structures, creating a high potential for false "negative" findings.

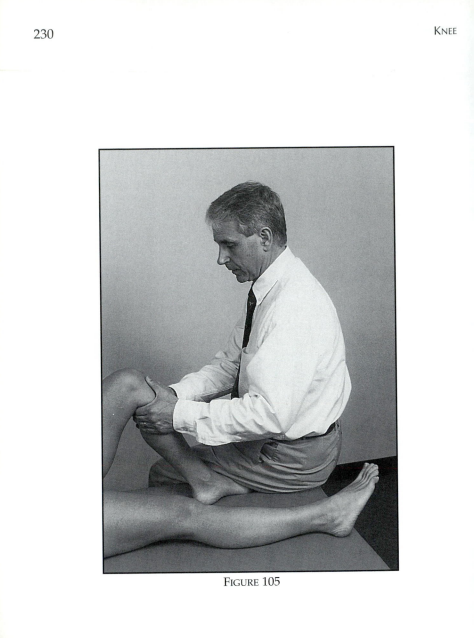

FIGURE 105

Pivot Shift Test

TEST POSITIONING:
The subject is supine with the test knee in full extension. The examiner is standing with the proximal hand on the subject's anterolateral tibio-femoral joint with the thumb on or posterior to the fibular head and the distal hand grasping the subject's midfoot and heel (Figure 106A). Alternate Test Positioning: Place the subject's foot between the examiner's distal arm and body with the same hand on the tibia, and the proximal hand on the posterolateral leg just distal to the knee with the thumb on or posterior to the fibular head.

ACTION:
Internally rotate the tibia with the distal hand, apply a valgus force with the proximal hand, and slowly flex the knee (Figure 106B). The same procedure applies for the alternate test positioning except first apply a slight axial load to the extended knee.

POSITIVE FINDING:
A palpable "clunk" or shift at ~20 to 30 degrees of flexion is indicative of anterolateral rotary instability, secondary to tearing of the ACL and posterolateral capsule.

SPECIAL CONSIDERATIONS/COMMENTS:
It is important to provide the axial load before flexing the knee, as this helps to accentuate the "clunk" or shift which will facilitate detection of a trace pivot shift. It should be noted that this test often reproduces the mechanism of injury which may create subject anxiety and apprehension, thus increasing the potential for false negative findings.

KNEE

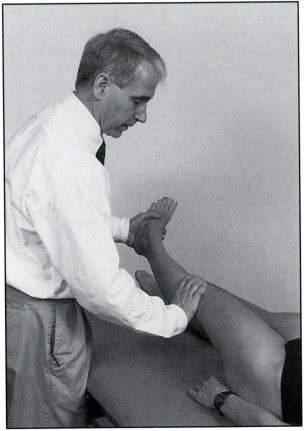

FIGURE 106A

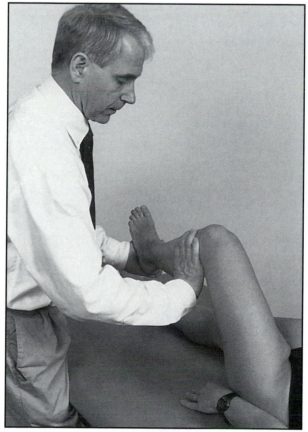

FIGURE 106B

Posterior Drawer Test

TEST POSITIONING:
The subject is supine with the test hip flexed to 45 degrees, knee flexed to 90 degrees, and foot in neutral position. The examiner is sitting on the subject's foot with both hands behind the subject's proximal tibia and thumbs on the tibial plateau (Figure 107).

ACTION:
Apply a posterior force to the proximal tibia.

POSITIVE FINDING:
Increased posterior tibial displacement as compared to the uninvolved side is indicative of a partial or complete tear of the PCL.

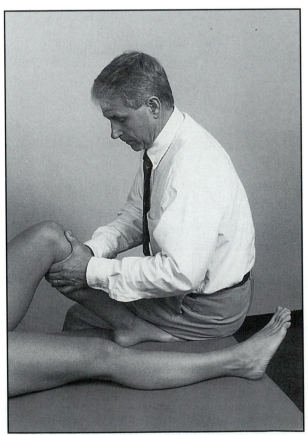

FIGURE 107

Hughston Posteromedial Drawer Test

TEST POSITIONING:
The subject is supine with the test hip flexed to 45 degrees, knee flexed to 90 degrees, and tibia internally rotated 20 to 30 degrees. The examiner is sitting on the subject's foot, with both hands behind the subject's proximal tibia and thumbs on the tibial plateau (Figure 108).

ACTION:
Apply a posterior force to the proximal tibia.

POSITIVE FINDING:
Increased posterior tibial displacement, particularly of the medial tibial condyle, as compared to the uninvolved side is indicative of posteromedial rotary instability, secondary to damage of primarily the PCL, posteromedial capsule, MCL, and posterior oblique ligament.

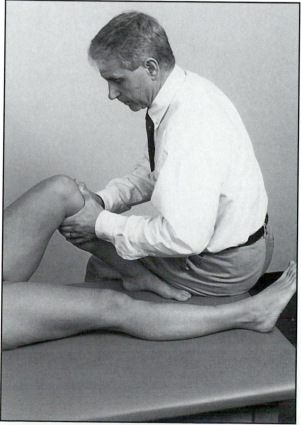

FIGURE 108

Hughston Posterolateral Drawer Test

TEST POSITIONING:
The subject is supine with the test hip flexed to 45 degrees, knee flexed to 90 degrees, and tibia externally rotated 20 to 30 degrees. The examiner is sitting on the subject's foot, with both hands behind the subject's proximal tibia and thumbs on the tibial plateau (Figure 109).

ACTION:
Apply a posterior force to the proximal tibia.

POSITIVE FINDING:
Increased posterior tibial displacement, particularly of the lateral tibial condyle, as compared to the uninvolved side is indicative of posterolateral rotary instability, secondary to damage of the PCL, LCL, posterolateral capsule, and arcuate complex.

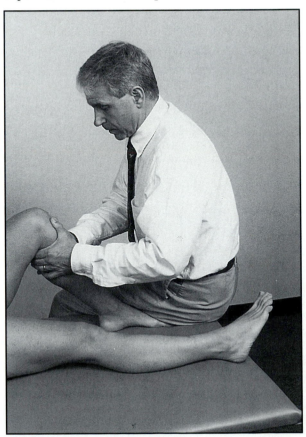

FIGURE 109

Posterior Lachman Test

TEST POSITIONING:
The subject is supine with the test knee flexed to 20 to 30 degrees. The examiner is standing with the proximal hand on the subject's distal thigh (laterally) just proximal to the patella, and the distal hand on the subject's proximal tibia (medially) just distal to the tibial tubercle (Figure 110).

ACTION:
From a "neutral" (anterior-posterior) position, apply a posterior force to the tibia with the distal hand while the femur is stabilized with the proximal hand.

POSITIVE FINDING:
Excessive posterior translation of the tibia (as compared to the uninvolved knee) from the neutral position with a diminished or absent endpoint is indicative of a partial or complete tear of the posterior cruciate ligament.

SPECIAL CONSIDERATIONS/COMMENTS:
If the Posterior Lachman Test is not performed from a neutral position, the involved knee may actually present with decreased posterior tibial translation as compared to the uninvolved knee. This decrease is most likely due to PCL pathology which allows the proximal tibia to translate posteriorly, thus producing decreased posterior translation and subsequent false negative findings. Therefore, the presence and quality of the endpoint must be determined before PCL integrity may be accurately assessed.

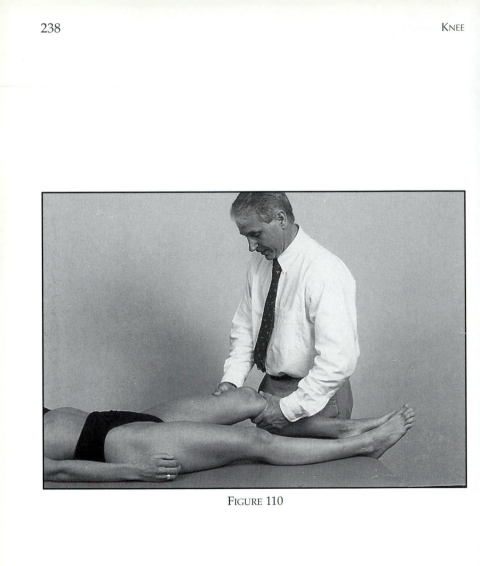

FIGURE 110

External Rotation Recurvatum Test

TEST POSITIONING:
The subject is supine. The examiner is standing and grasping a great toe with each hand.

ACTION:
Lift both legs off the table (vertically) by the great toes (Figure 111).

POSITIVE FINDING:
An increase in hyperextension and external tibial rotation as compared to the uninvolved knee is indicative of posterolateral rotary instability, secondary to damage of primarily the PCL, LCL, posterolateral capsule, and arcuate complex.

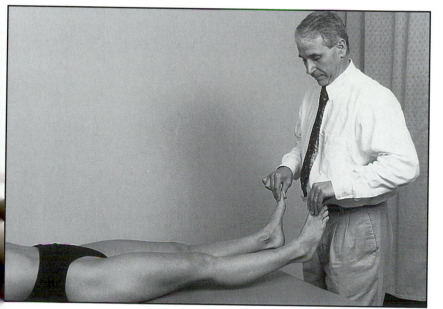

FIGURE 111

Valgus Stress Test

TEST POSITIONING:
The subject is supine with the knee in full extension (Figure 112A). The subject is supine with the knee in 20 to 30 degrees of flexion (Figure 112B). The examiner is standing with the distal hand on the subject's medial ankle and the proximal hand on the knee (laterally).

ACTION:
With the ankle stabilized, apply a valgus force at the knee with the proximal hand.

POSITIVE FINDING:
Medial knee pain and/or increased valgus movement with diminished or absent endpoint as compared to the uninvolved knee is indicative of damage to primarily the MCL, PCL, and posteromedial capsule in full extension and MCL in 20 to 30 degrees of flexion.

SPECIAL CONSIDERATIONS/COMMENTS:
The examiner must avoid allowing the femur to internally rotate during this test as this will give the illusion of increased valgus movement. This may be accomplished by using the treatment table to help stabilize the subject's femur.

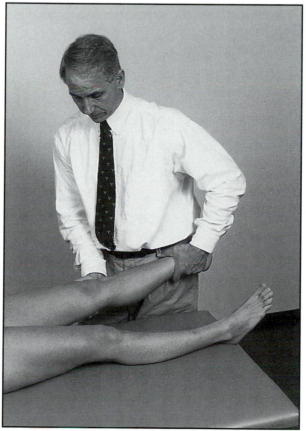

FIGURE 112A

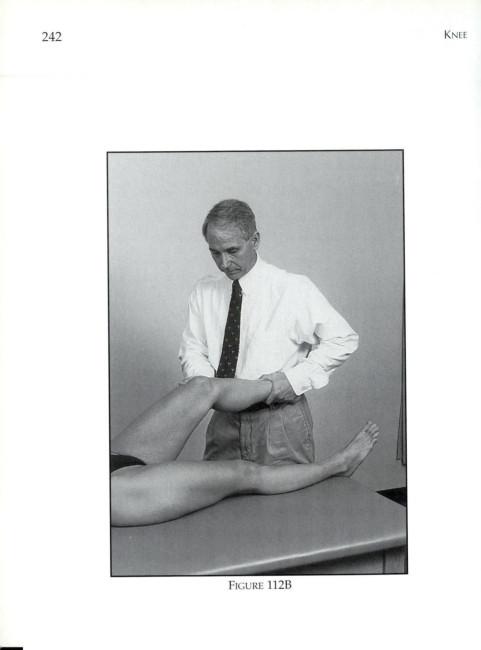

FIGURE 112B

Varus Stress Test

TEST POSITIONING:
The subject is supine with the knee in full extension (Figure 113A). The subject is supine with the knee in 20 to 30 degrees of flexion (Figure 113B). The examiner is standing with the distal hand on the subject's lateral ankle and the proximal hand on the knee (medially).

ACTION:
With the ankle stabilized, apply a varus force at the knee with the proximal hand.

POSITIVE FINDING:
Lateral knee pain and/or increased varus movement with diminished or absent endpoint as compared to the uninvolved knee is indicative of damage to primarily the LCL, PCL, and arcuate complex at 0 degrees of flexion and LCL at 20 to 30 degrees of flexion.

SPECIAL CONSIDERATIONS/COMMENTS:
The examiner must avoid allowing the femur to externally rotate during this test as this will give the illusion of increased varus movement. This may be accomplished by using the treatment table to help stabilize the subject's femur.

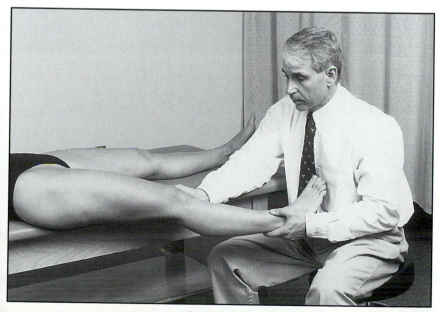

KNEE

FIGURE 113A

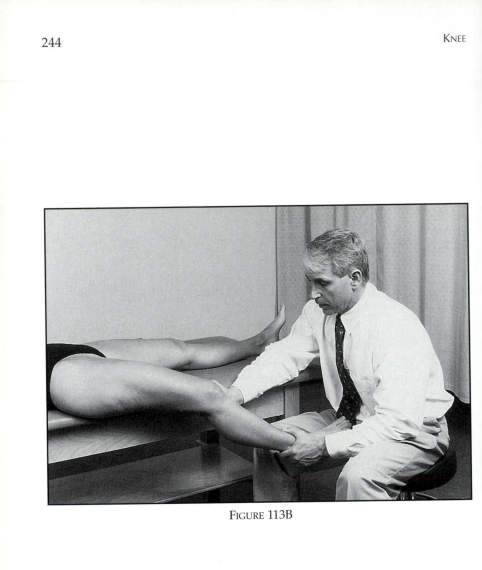

FIGURE 113B

Jerk Test

TEST POSITIONING:
The subject is lying supine with the involved hip flexed to 45 degrees. The examiner stands next to the involved side and holds the subject's foot. The examiner's other hand is placed over the lateral aspect of the knee, just behind the head of the fibula (Figure 114A).

ACTION:
The examiner passively flexes the subject's knee to 90 degrees (Figure 114B), then extends the subject's knee while applying valgus force and internally rotating the tibia (Figure 114C).

POSITIVE FINDING:
If a shift or clunk is felt at 30 degrees of knee flexion while the knee is being extended, a positive test is indicated, implicating anterolateral rotary instability. If a shift is present it will reduce upon further passive extension of the knee.

SPECIAL CONSIDERATIONS/COMMENTS:
This test may not be as sensitive as the Pivot Shift Test.

KNEE

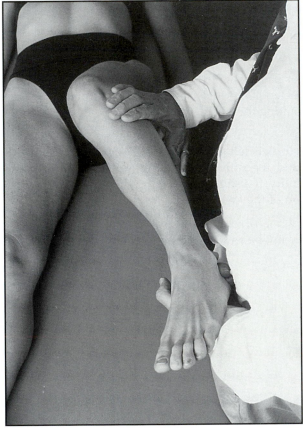

FIGURE 114A

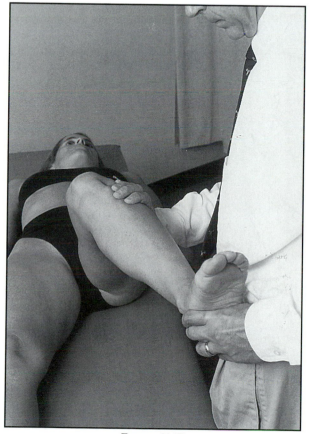

FIGURE 114B

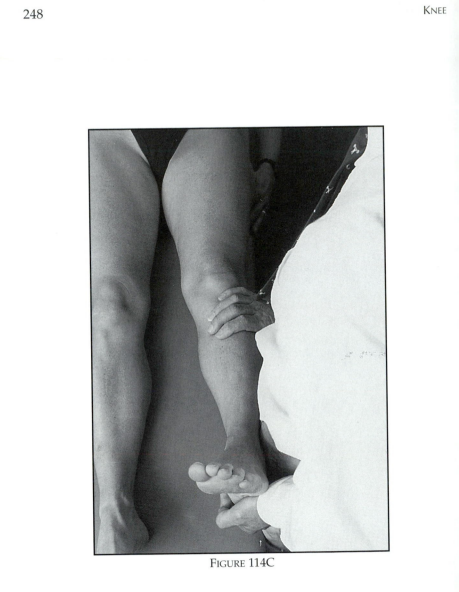

FIGURE 114C

McMurray Test

TEST POSITIONING:
The subject is supine. The examiner is standing with the distal hand grasping the subject's heel or distal leg (medially), and the proximal hand on the subject's knee with the fingers palpating the medial and lateral joint lines (Figure 115A).

ACTION:
With the knee fully flexed, externally rotate the tibia, introduce a valgus force, and extend the knee (medial meniscus) (Figure 115B). Repeat with the tibia internally rotated and a varus force applied to the knee (lateral meniscus) (Figure 115C).

POSITIVE FINDING:
A "click" along the medial joint line is indicative of a medial meniscus tear. Likewise, a "click" along the lateral joint line is indicative of a lateral meniscus tear.

SPECIAL CONSIDERATIONS/COMMENTS:
The examiner must not mistake a patellar "click" or "pop" for meniscal pathology.

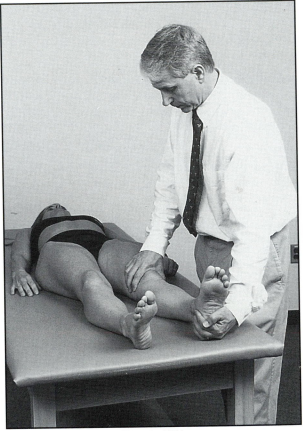

FIGURE 115A

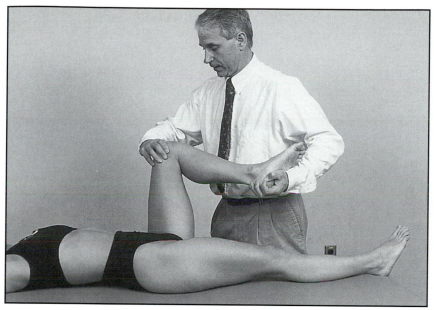

Figure 115B

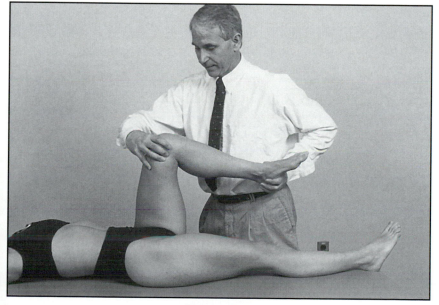

Figure 115C

Apley Compression Test

TEST POSITIONING:
The subject is prone with the test knee flexed to 90 degrees. The examiner is standing with the proximal hand on the subject's distal thigh for stabilization and the distal hand on the subject's heel (Figure 116A).

ACTION:
With the distal hand, medially and laterally rotate the tibia while applying a downward force through the heel.

POSITIVE FINDING:
Pain, clicking, and/or restriction is indicative of either a medial or lateral meniscus tear, depending on the location of symptoms.

SPECIAL CONSIDERATIONS/COMMENTS:
The test may be repeated with a distraction force (Apley Distraction Test) applied to the ankle with the distal hand (Figure 116B). An increase in and/or change in location of pain is more indicative of ligamentous versus meniscal pathology.

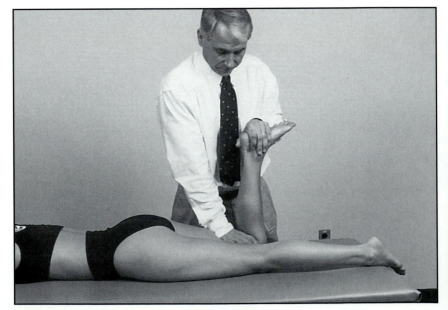

FIGURE 116A

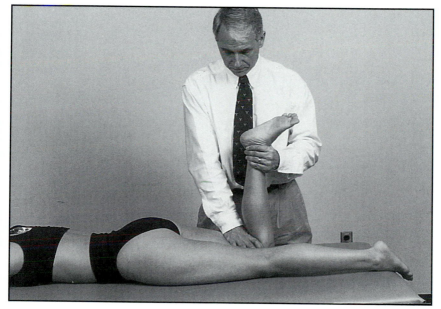

FIGURE 116B

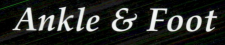

SECTION XII

Ankle & Foot

ANKLE & FOOT

Homan's Sign

TEST POSITIONING:
The subject lies supine on a table.

ACTION:
With the knee of the involved side fully extended, the examiner passively dorsiflexes the subject's foot (Figure 117A).

POSITIVE FINDING:
A production of pain in the calf that is brought upon by the passive stretch of the foot into a dorsiflexed position is a positive sign for thrombophlebitis.

SPECIAL CONSIDERATIONS/COMMENTS:
Pain may also be elicited upon palpation of the calf in conjunction with the passive stretch (Figure 117B). A positive finding indicates a life-threatening condition that should be addressed by appropriate medical personnel immediately.

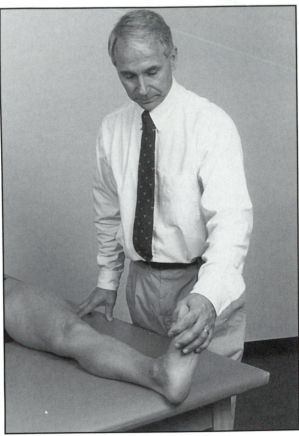

FIGURE 117A

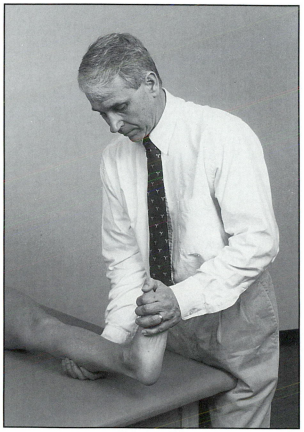

FIGURE 117B

Anterior Drawer Test

TEST POSITIONING:
The subject is seated on a table with the knee flexed to 90 degrees and the involved foot relaxed in slight plantar flexion. The examiner stabilizes the tibia and fibula with one hand and grasps the calcaneus with the other (Figure 118A). This may also be performed with the subject in a prone position (Figure 118B).

ACTION:
While assuring stabilization of the distal tibia and fibula, the examiner applies an anterior force to the calcaneus and talus.

POSITIVE FINDING:
Anterior translation of the talus away from the ankle mortise that is greater on the involved side, as opposed to the noninvolved side, indicates a positive sign for a possible anterior talofibular ligament sprain.

SPECIAL CONSIDERATIONS/COMMENTS:
The knee is flexed to 90 degrees to reduce the tension on the gastrocnemius muscle. This test should be performed bilaterally for comparison. Swelling within the ankle joint may reduce the ability to translate the talus anteriorly.

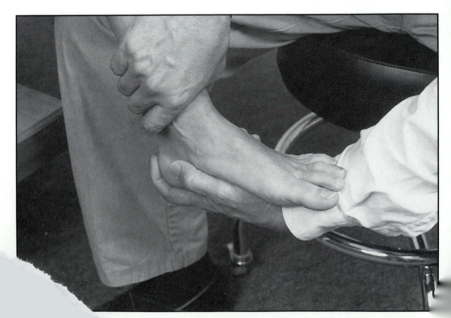

FIGURE 118A

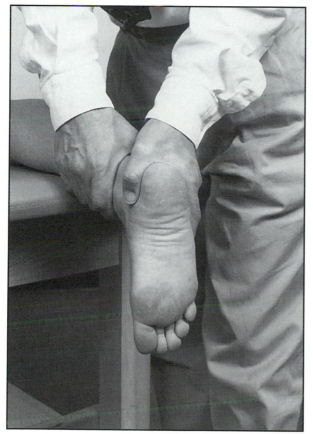

FIGURE 118B

Talar Tilt Test

TEST POSITIONING:

The subject is side lying (on the uninvolved side) on a table with the involved foot relaxed and the knee flexed to 90 degrees. The examiner stabilizes the distal tibia with one hand while grasping the talus with the other.

ACTION:

The examiner first places the foot in the anatomical position (neutral plantar and dorsiflexion). The examiner then tilts the talus into an adducted position (Figure 119).

POSITIVE FINDING:

Range of motion in the adducted position on the involved foot greater than that of the noninvolved foot reveals a positive test. This may be indicative for a tear of the calcaneofibular ligament of the ankle.

SPECIAL CONSIDERATIONS/COMMENTS:

The knee is flexed to 90 degrees to reduce the tension on the gastrocnemius muscle. This test should be performed bilaterally for comparison. Performing this test with the foot in a more plantar flexed position places less stress on the calcaneofibular ligament and instead may stress the anterior talofibular ligament. Swelling within the ankle joint may reduce the ability to translate the talus anteriorly.

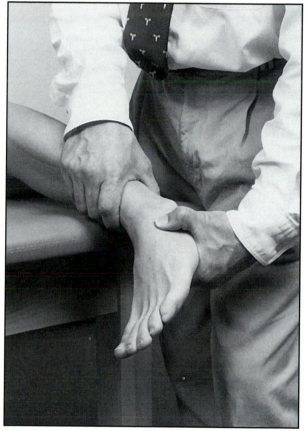

FIGURE 119

Thompson Test

TEST POSITIONING:
The subject lies prone on a table with the heels placed over the edge of the table.

ACTION:
With the gastrocnemius-soleus complex relaxed, the examiner squeezes the belly of these muscles (Figure 120).

POSITIVE FINDING:
When squeezing the calf muscles, a normal response would be to have the foot plantar flex. Therefore, an absence of plantar flexion upon squeezing would be a positive test, indicating a possible rupture of the achilles tendon.

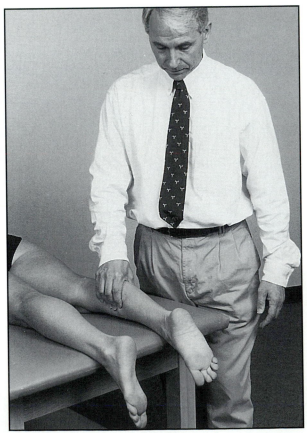

FIGURE 120

Tap or Percussion Test

TEST POSITIONING:
The subject is lying supine with the affected leg extended and the ankle/foot just off the examining table. The examiner stands at the end of the table next to the subject's foot.

ACTION:
The examiner positions the subject's ankle into maximal dorsiflexion, to optimize joint congruency, and applies a firm tap to the bottom of the subject's heel (Figure 121).

POSITIVE FINDING:
Pain at the site of injury is indicative of a fracture. The vibration of tapping along the long axis of the bones will exaggerate pain at the fracture site.

SPECIAL CONSIDERATIONS/COMMENTS:
This test should not be performed if there is obvious deformity.

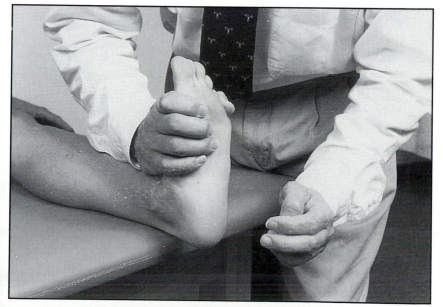

FIGURE 121

Feiss Line

TEST POSITIONING:
The subject is seated on the examining table with the involved leg extended. The examiner places a mark on the tip of the medial malleolus and at the base of the first metatarsophalangeal joint. A line is then drawn between the two points and the examiner notes the position of the navicular tuberosity (Figure 122A).

ACTION:
The subject is then asked to stand with feet 3 to 6 inches apart. The examiner ensures the marks are still positioned over the medial malleolus and first metatarsophalangeal joint, then again notes the position of the navicular tuberosity (Figure 122B).

POSITIVE FINDING:
The navicular tuberosity should be in line with the other two points. If while seated the navicular tuberosity is below the line, the subject has congenital pes planus. If while seated the navicular tuberosity is in line with the other two points, then falls below the line when the subject stands, functional pes planus is indicated.

SPECIAL CONSIDERATIONS/COMMENTS:
This test may be denotative of varying degrees of pes planus depending on how far the navicular drops to the floor. Pes planus may also be indicative of hyper-pronation.

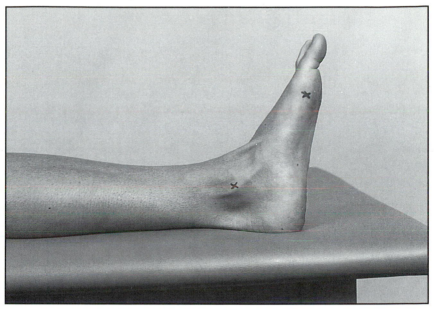

FIGURE 122A

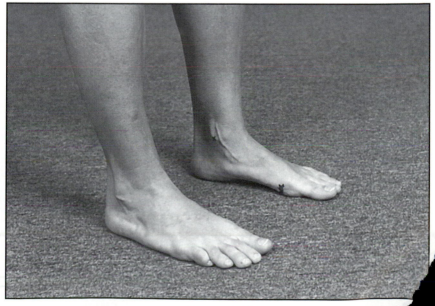

FIGURE 122B

Interdigital Neuroma Test

TEST POSITIONING:
The subject is seated on the examining table with the involved leg extended. The examiner stands next to the involved foot and places one hand around the metatarsal heads (Figure 123).

ACTION:
The examiner squeezes the subject's metatarsal heads together and holds for 1 to 2 minutes.

POSITIVE FINDING:
Pain, tingling, or numbness in the foot, toes, or ankle is indicative of an interdigital neuroma. If positive, pain is usually relieved when pressure is released.

SPECIAL CONSIDERATIONS/COMMENTS:
Pain between metatarsal heads is indicative of Morton's Neuroma. The most common location is between the third and fourth metatarsal heads.

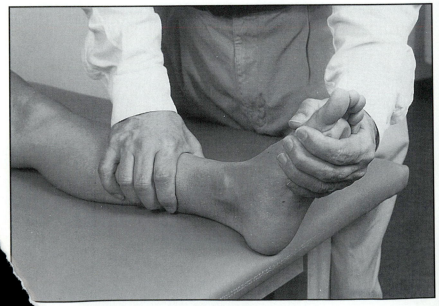

FIGURE 123

Compression Test

TEST POSITIONING:
The subject is lying supine with the affected leg extended and the ankle/foot just off the examining table. The examiner stands next to the subject's leg noting where the pain originates.

ACTION:
The examiner squeezes the tibia and fibula together at some point away from the painful area (Figure 124).

POSITIVE FINDING:
Pain at the site of injury may be indicative of a fracture. Compression of the two bones may exaggerate pain at the fracture site.

SPECIAL CONSIDERATIONS/COMMENTS:
This test should not be performed if there is obvious deformity. A positive test is not exclusive of a fracture. It is recommended that an X-ray always confirm suspicion of a fracture.

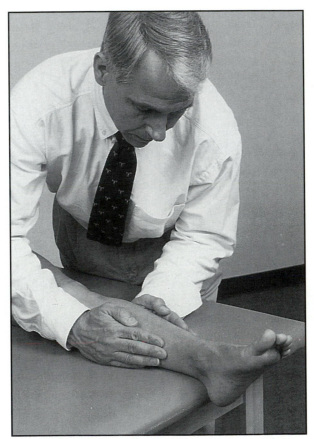

Figure 124

Long Bone Compression Test

TEST POSITIONING:
The subject is seated with the affected leg extended and the foot off the end of the examining table. The examiner stands at the end of the table near the subject's foot.

ACTION:
The examiner applies compression along the long axis of the bone of the toe or metatarsal being tested (Figure 125).

POSITIVE FINDING:
Pain at the site of injury is indicative of a fracture.

SPECIAL CONSIDERATIONS/COMMENTS:
This test should not be performed if there is obvious deformity.

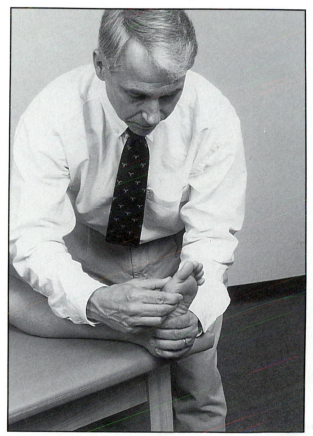

FIGURE 125

References

Adams MC. *Outline of Orthopaedics*. London: E & S Livingstone; 1968.

Anderson AF, Lipscomb AB. Clinical diagnosis of meniscal tears: Description of a new manipulative test. *Am J Sports Med*. 1988;14:291.

Andrews JR, Gillogly S. Physical examination of the shoulder in throwing athletes. In: Zarins BJ, Andrews JR, Carson WG, eds. *Injuries to the Throwing Arm*. Philadelphia, Pa: WB Saunders; 1985.

Archibald KC, Wiechec F. A Reappraisal of Hoover's test. *Arch Phys Med Rehabil*. 1970;51:234.

Arieff AJ, Tigay EI, Kurtz JF, Larmon WA. The hoover sign: An objective sign of pain and/or weakness in the back or lower extremities. *Arch Neurol*. 1961;5:673.

Aulcino PL, DuPuy TE. Clinical examination of the hand. In: Hunter J, et al. *Rehabilitation of the Hand: Surgery and Therapy*. St. Louis, Mo: CV Mosby; 1990.

Booher JM, Thibodeau GA. *Athletic Injury Assessment*. St. Louis, Mo: CV Mosby; 1994.

Brody IA, Williams RH. The signs of Kernig and Brudzinski. *Arch Neurol*. 1969;21:215.

Clarkson HM, Gilewich GB. *Musculoskeletal Assessment: Joint Range of Motion and Manual Muscle Strength*. Baltimore, Md: Williams & Wilkins; 1989.

Cram RH. A sign of sciatic nerve root pressure. *J Bone Joint Surg*. 1953;35B:192.

D'Alessandro DF, Valadie AL. Superior glenoid lesions: A diagnositc and therapeutic challenge. *J Southern Orthop Assoc*. 1995;4(3):214-227.

Gerber C, Ganz R. Clinical assessment of instability of the shoulder. *J Bone Joint Surg*. 1984;66B:551-556.

Gogia PP. *Clinical Orthopedic Tests: An Illustrated Reference*. Tucson, Az: Therapy Skill Builders; 1994.

Grubel-Lee DM. *Disorders of the Hip*. Philadelphia, Pa: JB Lippincott; 1983.

Hertling D, Kessler RM. *Management of Common Musculoskeletal Disorders: Physical Therapy Principles and Methods*. 2nd ed. Philadelphia, Pa: JB Lippincott; 1990.

Hoover CF. A new sign for the detection of malingering and functional paresis of the lower extremities. *JAMA*. 1908;51:746.

Hoppenfeld S. *Physical Examination of the Spine and Extremities*. Norwalk: Appleton-Century-Crofts; 1976.

Hughston JC, Walsh WM, Puddu G. *Patellar Subluxation and Dislocation*. Philadelphia, Pa: WB Saunders; 1984.

Jakob RP, Hassler H, Staeubli HU. Observations on rotary instability of the lateral compartment of the knee. *Acta Orthop Scand*. (Suppl. 191). 1981;52:1.

Magee DJ. *Orthopedic Physical Assessment*. 2nd ed. Philadelphia, Pa: WB Saunders; 1992.

Manzi, DB, Weaver, PA. *Head Injury: The Acute Care Phase*. Thorofare, NJ: Slack Inc; 1987.

Noble HS, Hajak MR, Portes M. Diagnosis and treatment of iliotibial band tightness in runners. *Physician and Sports Medicine*. 1982;10(4):67-74.

O'Riain S. Shrivel test: A new and simple test of nerve function in the hand. *Br Med J*. 1973;3:615.

Palmer ML, Epler M. *Clinical Assessment Procedures in Physical Therapy*. Philadelphia, Pa: JB Lippincott; 1990.

Post M. *Physical Examination of the Musculoskeletal System*. Chicago, Ill: Year Book Medical Publishing; 1987.

Renne JW. The iliotibial band friction syndrome. *J Bone Joint Surg.* 1975;57A(8):1110-1111.

Ruwe PA, et al. Clinical determination of femoral anteversion: A comparison with established techniques. *J Bone Joint Surg Am.* 1992;74:820.

Saunders HD, Saunders R. *Evaluation, Treatment and Prevention of Musculoskeletal Disorders.* 3rd ed. Volume 1-Spine. Bloomington, In: Educational Opportunities; 1993.

Scully RM, Barnes MR. *Physical Therapy.* Philadelphia, Pa: JB Lippincott; 1989.

Spengler DM. *Low Back Pain: Assessment and Management.* Orlando, Fla: Grune & Stratton; 1982.

Staheli, LT. Medial femoral torsion. *Orthop Clin North Am.* 1980;11:39.

Starkey C, Ryan JL. *Evaluation of Orthopedic and Athletic Injuries.* Philadelphia, Pa: FA Davis; 1996.

Strobel M, Stedtfeld HW. *Diagnostic Evaluation of the Knee.* Berlin: Springer-Verlag; 1990.

Taleisnik J. Carpal instability. *J Bone Joint Surg.* 1988;70A:1262-1268.

Thompson T, Doherty J. Spontaneous rupture of the tendon of Achilles: A new clinical diagnostic test. *Anat Res.* 1967;158:126.

Topel JL. Examination of the comatose patient. In: Weiner WJ, Goetz CG: *Neurology for the Non-Neurologist.* Philadelphia, Pa: JB Lippincott; 1989.

Walsh DA. Shoulder evaluation of the throwing athlete. *Sports Med Update.* 1989;4:24-27.

Yergason RM. Supination sign. *J Bone Joint Surg.* 1931;13:160.